To Paul,
Thank you
me market
tomorrow in the Rehoboth Half &
all your future trianthelons
Michael Scadron

Two Mountains:

Kilimanjaro to Quadriplegic and Back

S. Michael Scadron

Bethesda Communications Group

Published by the Bethesda Communications Group
4816 Montgomery Lane
Bethesda, MD 20814
www.bcgpub.com

ISBN-13: 978-1-7321501-0-2
ISBN-10: 1-7321501-0-9

The photos included are all from the Scadron family photos.

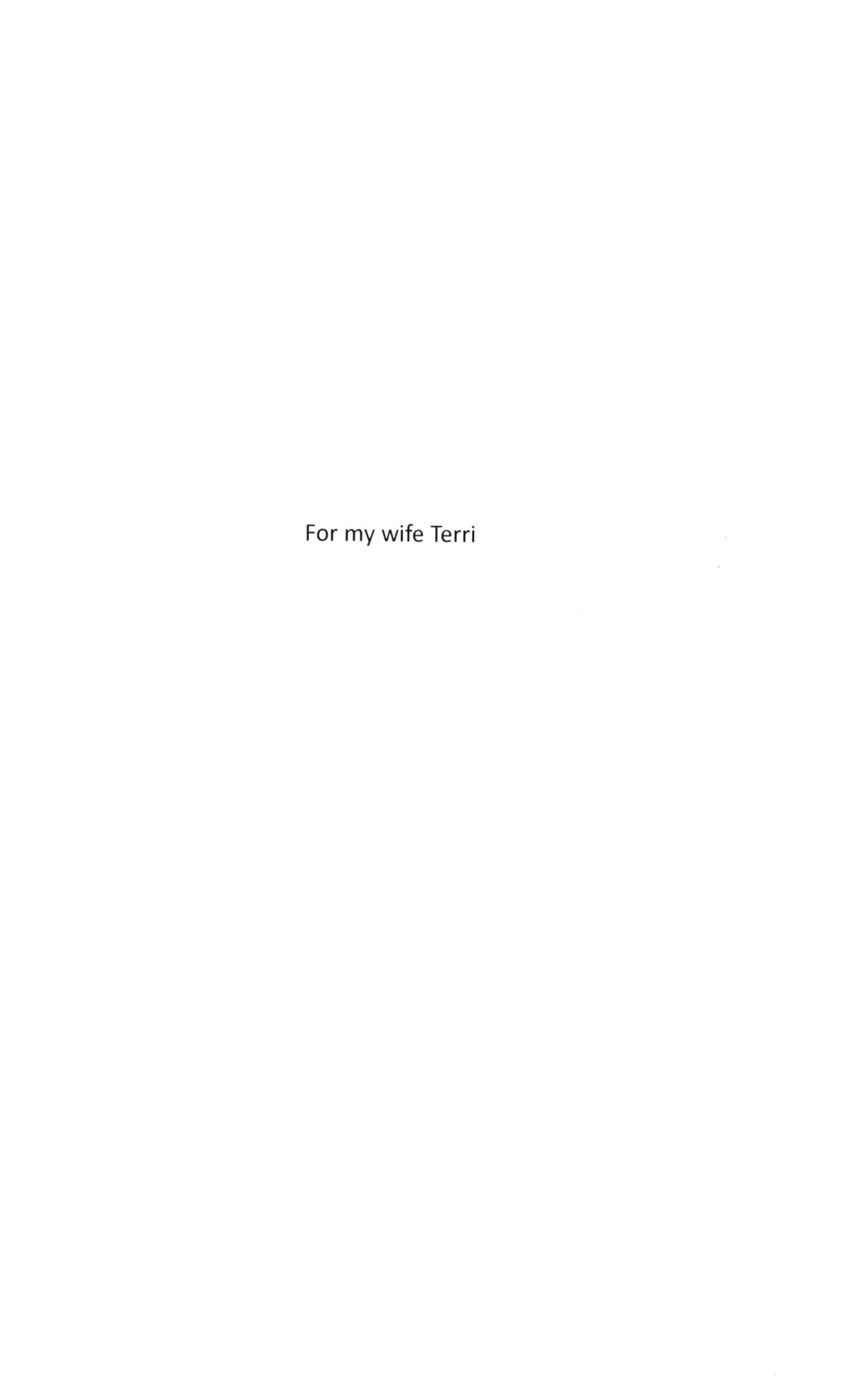

For my wife Terri

Contents

Acknowledgements

When I retired from the Justice Department in 2006, determined to take up writing as my new career, a colleague asked me plainly enough what I planned on writing about. Without hesitation, I told her that I wanted to write about legal cases that I found interesting, especially cases resulting in injustices. She said that I should consider writing about my medical condition, that my story of suddenly having to cope with a crippling illness just after turning 50 would inspire many folks struggling day to day with disability. I was skeptical. I was never interested in reading medical memoirs, much less writing one. But her suggestion planted a seed in my brain that grew as I studied creative non-fiction at the Bethesda Writers Center and engaged in writing workshops. After a couple of years, I'd produced a first draft that wasn't terribly exciting, but at least it laid out the myriad details that I might have forgotten had I waited much longer.

Feeling burnt out on the topic, I shelved the project for several years, turning my attention instead to travel articles, short personal essays, and articles about injustices at home and abroad. I'd put too much work into my medical memoir, however, to abandon it altogether. Eventually, I turned back to it, dispensing with the mundane and tedious parts while adding personal reflections and musings. I know that the end product is light years better than my early draft and hope that the work will, indeed, be of benefit to others facing adversity.

This memoir has been a work in progress for more than a decade and many people have helped me with critiques and advice along the way. I'd first like to thank my editor and publisher, Debbie Lange, for her interest in the book and her many thoughtful edits, particularly pointing out my overcrowded sentences (a lawyer's trait, I'm afraid). She has helped improve my work significantly.

I'd also like to thank Sara Taber, an author and instructor at the Bethesda Writers Center, for her thorough edits and wisdom in helping me struggle through my early draft. I owe a debt of gratitude to the many writers who attended Sara's workshop who were generous with their thoughts and comments.

As I've revised the book in recent years, I am grateful for the instructors and published authors who comprise my writers critique group for the time they've spent commenting and suggesting edits chapter by chapter. In this regard, I owe thanks to Bonny Miller, Diana Parsell, Cheryl LaRoche, Ken Ackerman, Judi Latte, Sonja Williams, Nancy Derr, and Michael Kirkland.

I owe special thanks to my friends, family, and work colleagues, including my daughter, Jessica, who suffered through my ordeal, supporting me throughout. Some of these folks make appearances in the book, and a number have been kind enough to pen tributes that I have included in my website at www.michaelscadron.com.

In writing about friends and family members, I've used first names only to preserve a modicum of privacy. Hopefully, they will forgive me for taking certain liberties in recreating scenes and dialogue. In doing so, I've tried to stay faithful to their respective traits and personalities, at least in so far as my own memories and perceptions allow.

Finally, I couldn't have made it this far without the unyielding help and support of my wife, Terri. This is apparent throughout the book. What is not apparent is that Terri won first place in the Bethesda Literary Festival in 2012 for her inspirational essay about our ordeal. It was published in *Bethesda Magazine* in July 2012. I have included Terri's essay, "Measured Steps," in my website under "Terri's View." See https://www.michaelscadron.com/terris-view/.

With publication of this book, I may have conquered my third mountain.

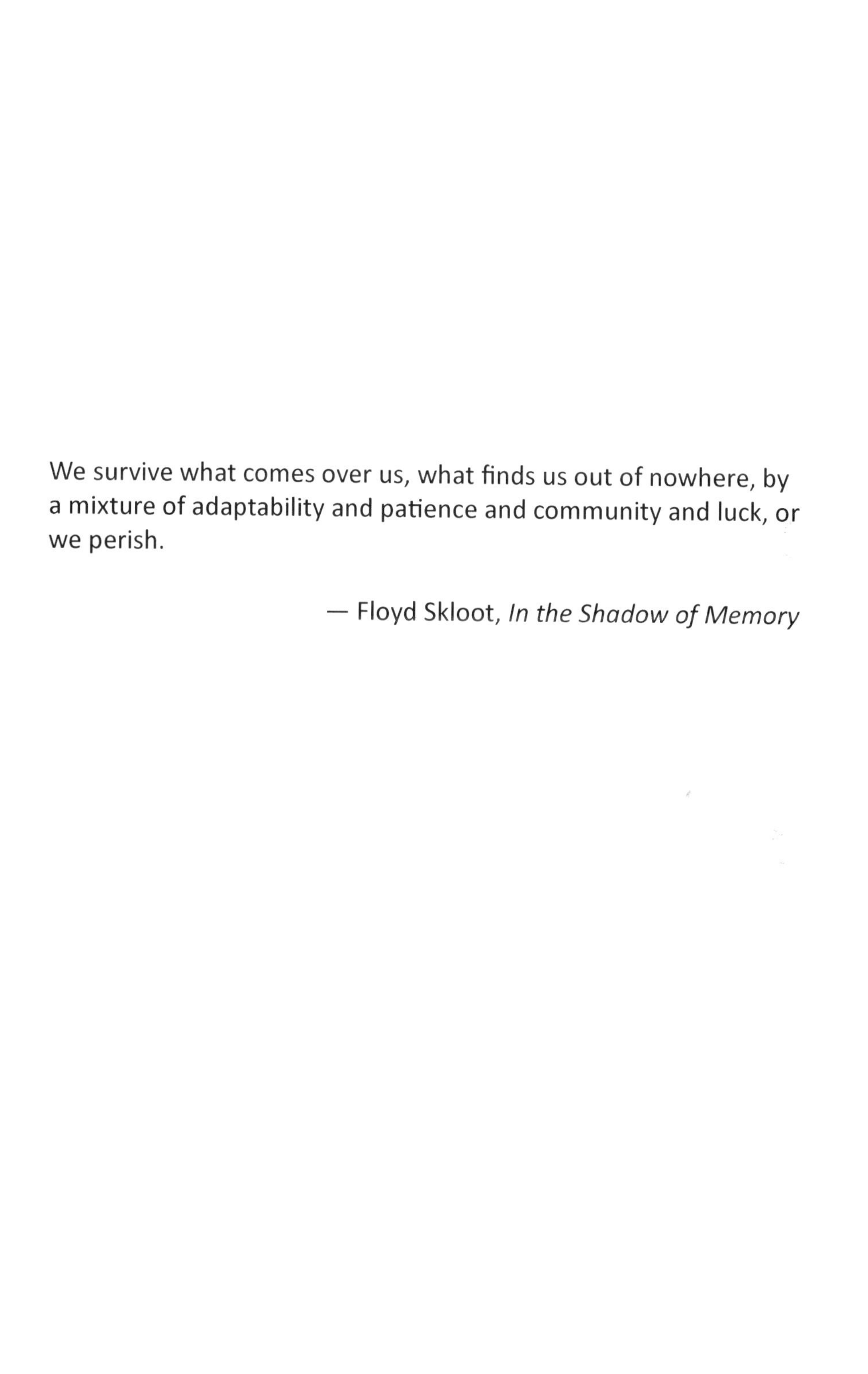

We survive what comes over us, what finds us out of nowhere, by a mixture of adaptability and patience and community and luck, or we perish.

— Floyd Skloot, *In the Shadow of Memory*

Part One: Falling

1 Ascending the Mountain

I'm perspiring as if I'd been jogging for five miles under a noonday sun. Billie, my physical therapist, removes my walker, tightens the safety belt she fastened around my waist, and helps me place my sweaty hands on the metal railings. She retrieves the talcum powder from my wife, Terri, and applies a generous amount to the left railing. My wife does the same for the opposite one. I'll need the firmest grip I can muster. I glance behind me. The evening concierge is watching from her perch at the front desk. My nerves are on edge as I look ahead toward the same five steps I've been struggling to conquer for several months now.

It was November 2000—one year since I first knew something was wrong with me, and six months since I got out of the hospital, crippled by an immune-related neuropathy that weakened me mysteriously, gradually, before striking with a vengeance and rendering me quadriplegic. Since then I'd been wedded to a wheelchair, relying on Terri to guide me through each day.

Terri and I had been together for less than three years before my illness struck. My marriage to her was my second. An earlier marriage to a tormented artist ended in divorce, followed soon after by her death from brain cancer. I was then thrust into the role of Mr. Mom to my seven-year-old daughter, Jessica. Terri entered the picture when Jessica turned 15. Terri and I became soul mates before my illness; after it we were inseparable.

Second time around made for a wiser choice. And it would be an unendurable agony to face this all by myself.

Terri accompanied me to all of my medical appointments and most of my therapy sessions with Billie. Billie was a middle-aged Ugandan woman. Soft spoken, yet mercilessly persistent, she came to our uptown Connecticut Avenue apartment in D.C. Tuesdays and Thursdays at seven in the evening. This schedule, put in place after my release from the hospital in May 2000, afforded my wife and me time to drive home from work once I was able to work. It was fortunate that we worked in the same downtown office building. I could no longer drive myself.

Slender, of medium height, and fashionably dressed, Billie had been working with me ever since my homecoming—weights, balancing exercises, indoor walks with my walker and safety belt, or whatever she could conjure up to challenge me. In September, despite much effort but little progress on my part, she decided it was time for me to tackle stairs.

"I can't do them," I said, "but if you want to, I'm happy to watch." I have a lifelong habit of using humor to mask my inner dread. Billie smiled, but didn't miss a beat.

"I'll help, but I think you are ready to try stairs."

"You'll rise to the occasion," Terri said, unable to mask a sly smile.

Billie, Terri and I, with the help of my walker, took the elevator to the lobby. We approached the steps leading from the main lobby up to the landing and the street entrance. I counted five of them, not steep and fairly wide with metal railings on either side. I'd scurried up and down these stairs without a moment's thought for the 12 years I'd lived in this high-rise condominium. I'd never before had reason to count them.

With a slight boost from Billie, who had one hand lightly on my safety belt, I managed to place my left leg on the first step, but I couldn't get my other leg to join it. My shirt collar was soaked from perspiration and my hands slipped on the railings. Mercifully, Billie called an end to that first session and asked Terri to buy talcum powder to use the next time.

The use of the powder solved the problem of my grip on the

railings, but it took several sessions before I could coax my right leg to join my left on the first step, and many more before I could do it without a boost from Billie.

Now, as I approach the stairway for the umpteenth time, I'm yearning to make it all the way to the top. Uh oh, there's Mrs. Burton returning home from some volunteer meeting. I'll wait for her to shuffle down the other side of the steps. The presence of onlookers unnerves me. I hate appearing like a freak in a circus sideshow. She smiles. I look away. Just focus. I look down at the first step. Time to move. First my left leg, then my right leg, and then a little rest.

I feel Billie's hand on my back. I hate this. If I have to climb these steps, I'll damn well do it without a push or a nudge. "Don't give me a boost, Billie. If I'm going to do this it has to be all on my own."

"I'm not boosting you; I just have one hand lightly on the belt."

Now the second step. Left leg, then right. Slow and steady. One step at a time. I pause before tackling the third step. Left leg, then right. Three steps completed and two to go. The top landing is now within my grasp. Just two more steps.

My thoughts meander to a time, not long ago, when I was fit and healthy, to the trip Terri and I took to East Africa the summer before last, to our successful ascent to the summit of Kilimanjaro.

It was getting late and James, our husky no-nonsense guide, was anxious to get going. He asked each of us—Terri and me, and our climbing companions, Ray and Lisa—whether we were ready for the final push. "Alright then, turn your headlamps on." But our headlamps, fastened like bandanas around our foreheads, wouldn't go on, or we couldn't figure out how to get them to work. Not a great way to start out.

Terri fiddled with hers. She shook it, turned it sideways, and tried just about everything, to no avail. "We just bought them brand new at Hudson Trail Outfitters up the street from us. I suppose we should have seen if they worked. We don't have time to mess with them now."

Ray's headlamp and Lisa's were flickering and they too eventually went dead. "Maybe it's the altitude," I said.

James sighed in frustration.

We knew what he was thinking. Dumb tourists.

"Follow me," he said. "We'll have to make do with my flashlight and the moon. Stay close." It was eleven at night, and we'd rested for only a few hours.

We'd trekked for five days through rainforest, across alpine meadow, through the moonscape above the tree line. Then, the final ascent, all night until morning, over loose pebbles, snow and ice. At 19,000 feet, snow-capped Kilimanjaro is the tallest freestanding mountain in the world.

James planned for us to begin our march to the summit at eleven at night with the hopes of arriving by eight or so in the morning, before the snow got too soft. We'd camped at 15,500 feet where sleep had been out of the question for me. Terri can sleep any time, anywhere. I just lay in my tent, hoping a few hours rest would be enough to carry me through what we knew would be an ordeal.

When James announced that we were to begin, I had quickly donned my layers of long underwear, ski pants, ski jacket, and hat, all of which I'd borrowed from a friend who was experienced at this outdoor stuff. The outer ski clothing fit too tightly for comfort, but would have to suffice. With any luck I wouldn't have to take a whiz.

We maneuvered slowly by moonlight, trudging along for what seemed an eternity, first one foot, then the other, one step at a time. If any one of us felt symptoms of altitude sickness, such as a headache, we'd have to descend. No sense in risking serious health consequences. We had with us diamox, an oral medicine prescribed to reduce symptoms of altitude sickness. Thankfully, Terri seemed okay having taken it the night before.

By daybreak we could see the sunrise over Malawi, the second highest of Kilimanjaro's three peaks. A sliver of sun peeking out over a sea of ruffled clouds outlined the sharp contours of the charcoal dome bathing it in a golden hue. A splendid sight, though

James told us we still had three hours before we could expect to reach the summit crater on Kibo, the highest peak, "the roof of Africa."

We'd begun our ascent walking on loose pebbles, circling rocks and boulders. Now, there was hard, packed snow and ice all around. We progressed at an even slower pace, having to stop and rest by leaning on our ski poles, taking deep breaths after every step. No one spoke; to do so would waste needed energy. The temperature was well below freezing, and our water bottles were solid blocks of ice. We were lucky the wind was light. The ice glistened as the intense equatorial sun gained stature.

I began to stop for two deep breaths between each step. I wasn't physically exhausted yet, but the air was thin and my breathing more labored. Plus, I knew this was a safe pace. We'd been told to pace ourselves so that we'd never be out of breath. "Exaggerate your breathing," James had said.

Like a scuba diver who must ascend slowly to avoid "the bends," I was keenly aware that a slow ascent was far safer than a speedy one. This way, we wouldn't exhaust ourselves prematurely, causing pulmonary or cerebral edema.

Soon I needed a longer rest. Although the air was frigid, perspiration dripped down my forehead and neck. I looked back to see Terri struggling, then leaned on my pole and sucked in the cold thin air. Breathe in, breathe out. I strained to see how far we had left to go. Hard to tell. Could the summit be that much further? How long have we been at this? Seven hours? Eight maybe. And the long, slippery trek down the mountain still lay ahead with no thought of sleep before nightfall. What in heavens name did we get ourselves into? Walking up steep slopes for nine hours on no sleep, knowing we'd have to go back down for another nine hours. Were we crazy?

After a few minutes I saw Terri making slow but steady progress. Good Luck, James' aptly named assistant guide, was helping her, so I resumed my climb. Finally, by 8:30 am, we reached the crater. First Ray, then Lisa, then me—we staggered to the top. Finally Terri, still in the company of Good Luck, crawled her way up the last few hundred meters.

The clouds swirled around us diminishing visibility toward the two-mile wide summit crater. Breaks in the clouds on the side we had climbed, however, allowed for a view of the grassy, acacia-studded plains of Africa below.

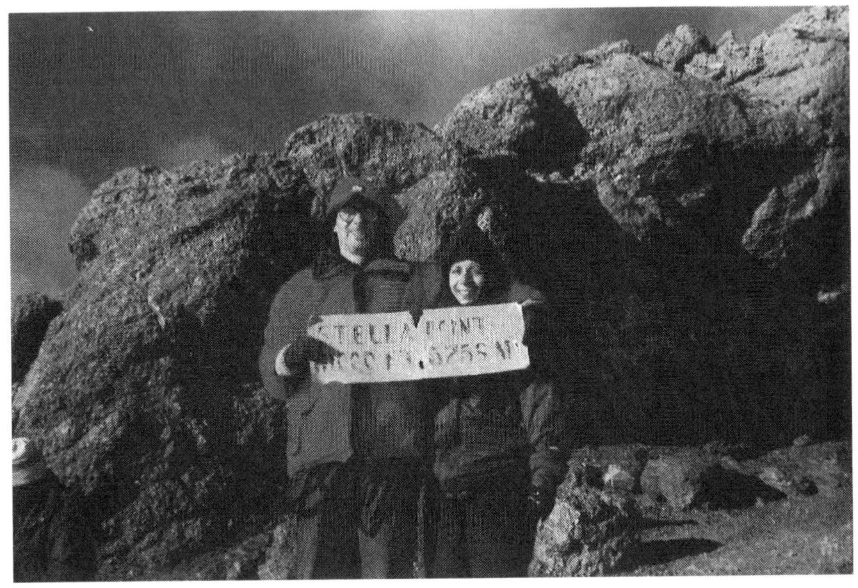

Terri and Michael, having reached the summit
of Kilimanjaro, 5758 meters (19,000 feet)

I took two deep breaths and looked around. After five exhausting days, here we were on the roof of Africa. Exhilaration swept over my spent body. I was Frank Shorter winning the Olympic marathon, Muhammad Ali knocking out Joe Frazier. I was the man who broke the bank at Monte Carlo. We would descend to a hero's welcome, like Edmund Hillary and his Sherpa, Tenzing Norgay, the first mountaineers to successfully climb Everest, returning to glory.

Now hold it right there, I told myself, you're getting a little too full of yourself and giddy, maybe from the altitude. Thousands of others have done this haven't they, but still.... I thought about Hemingway and the frozen carcass of a leopard found near the top of the mountain. What had that leopard been seeking at such high altitude, Hemingway had asked. What was it that we were seeking? A sense of accomplishment perhaps, but more than that for me. Growing up in New York City, and at summer camp as a youngster, I'd always spurned athletics. Those who knew me then would never think I'd be capable of a feat like this. Thus, for me there was some redemption in this achievement, a rebellion of sorts against my sheltered childhood.

In more recent times, I'd accomplished some worthy feats, like running the ten-mile Cherry Blossom in under seventy-five minutes after turning 50. Even so, this was harder than anything physical I'd ever done, something I could rightfully be proud of. But not boastful, I'd have to be careful about that. Athletic accomplishments aside, my life was pretty darn good. I'd recently won a big case as a trial lawyer at the Justice Department and had developed a fine reputation there. And marrying Terri was a true blessing. Yes, life was good, maybe too good.

James interrupted my reverie. "We have a long walk ahead," he said. "Take in the view, have a little rest, and then we must start down." He pointed to his watch. "Fifteen minutes."

After snapping some photos, taking in the scenery, and then resting, we began the long scramble down the mountain. I cherish the photo Ray took of Terri and me smiling and holding the sign left for us by other climbers. It designated the altitude at the spot where we had reached the summit to be 5,758 meters (19,000 feet).

Now, as I tackle the final two steps to the landing above the condo lobby, it occurs to me that going down will be trickier than going up. Yet, as with any mountain, I cannot claim success until I return to base camp safely. Just gotta do it. This is not the time to chicken out. Focus.

Billie brings the walker up to me. I'll have to step into it and turn around with it toward the stairs, then push it aside before I reach down to grip the railings. They're awfully low—I'll have to bend my knees. This would be easy enough if my muscles were working. They aren't. If I bend my knees too much they'll buckle and I'll go down. I feel like a novice skier who must jump from the ski lift, and immediately start skiing back downhill. The top part of my shirt is soaked with sweat.

I tell myself to ignore the comings and goings of the condo residents. Can't afford the luxury of feeling self-conscious. Just focus. I hesitate at the top of the stairs for an eternity. Billie is standing behind me holding my safety belt. "You can't stand here all night."

Terri positions herself alongside me for moral support. "Just another rock scramble, like Kilimanjaro."

As my past life flashes before me, I bend my knees. But I hold firm, maneuvering my legs down just as I had coaxed them upward—one step at a time. I can do this. Bend the knees. Right leg, left leg. Success at last.

The concierge applauds from her place behind the desk. I feel relief coupled with a sense of achievement. Terri mops the perspiration from my brow.

"Now it's Miller time," I suggest to all who can hear.

"Not quite yet," Billie says. "After a little rest, we have more exercises to do. Then you may have your happy hour."

Slave driver.

Miracle worker.

I recall the time when Terri, Ray, Lisa, and I had completed our descent of Kilimanjaro and stopped at the village at the gateway to the trail so we could buy the porters beers and toast our accomplishment. Beer or not, like then, I'm feeling sky high.

2 Falling

The first omen came when I embarked on my usual long run, a seven-mile loop through Rock Creek Park. The park drive leads from a residential street just east of the Cleveland Park neighborhood of Washington, D.C., where I then lived, and winds uphill for about one-half mile to the high road near a public horse stable. Ordinarily I looked forward to the challenge of this hill. I started out with mental energy that I needed to unleash. But as I labored up the hill I felt my legs grow tight. Maybe, I thought, when I reach the top and the road levels off, perhaps then my body will loosen up. I rounded the bend where the trees on the right side give way to a green expanse occupied by a horse paddock and trails. "Run," I told myself, but my legs didn't respond. I felt unusually sluggish, like I'd just run a long distance road race the day before, although I hadn't. Frustrated, and confused about my sluggishness, I slowed my pace to a jog.

It was late November 1999, just after the Thanksgiving holiday. I was 52 years old, a trial lawyer with the Justice Department for most of my career, and had almost never been sick in my life. My only hospitalization had been to have my tonsils out when I was four.

Just a few months earlier, in late July, Terri and I had completed our trek to the summit of Mount Kilimanjaro. I savored this feat, even bragged about it to all who could bear to listen, because

I'd never been particularly athletic. All my life I'd lacked the coordination and fluidity of movement required for success at most sports. The big exception was running, which simply required dogged determination. But nothing in my past would have suggested that I'd ever willingly take on the challenge of tackling a serious mountain.

I grew up in an apartment on Manhattan's upper west side with my aggressively sedentary extended family. Neither my mother, who we called Sis, nor my Aunt Ceal, nor my older cousins, Patsy and Judy, would walk more than two blocks if they could take a taxi. I became a rebel of sorts. I took up running after law school and spent my lunch hours jogging on the Mall. Herds of Government workers can be seen running mid-day on the National Mall or circling the city's fabled marbled monuments.

I'd run with my colleague, Kevin, who was an ultra-marathoner. He'd commute from his home in Great Falls, Virginia, by running the 12 miles back and forth to our downtown offices. In between he'd take the time to accompany me on my four or five mile lunch hour jog (I'd sometimes find him dozing off mid-afternoon). Before long, due to Kevin's tutelage, I was running much faster than before.

I ran obsessively every day in the years that followed. When I was nearing fifty I started running in 10K road races with a small circle of friends. Who would have thought that I, so uninterested in sports most of my young life, would become so competitive?

Though never the athlete, you couldn't say I wasn't fit. So when the budding notion of climbing Kilimanjaro took hold, such an endeavor didn't seem so daunting. There'd be no specialized mountaineering skills required, only that one be able to place one foot in front of another, be in good enough condition to tackle steep slopes for several days, brave occasional rock scrambles, and, most important, be willing to persevere. So, what the heck?

The tightness in my legs I'd first noticed shortly after Thanksgiving continued for the next several weeks. For most of December I didn't seem to be getting worse, at least not that I could tell. Probably just a passing affliction that would cure itself in time. No way could I have guessed that I was in the early stages of a crippling neurological condition that would require me to tackle a mountain far more challenging than the one I had conquered a short while back.

For New Year's week, Terri, Jessica, and I went to visit friends in Vero Beach, Florida. By then, I was noticing numbness in my feet and my balance was slightly off. We were staying just across the inland waterway, about a mile or so from the beach, and the bridge crossing the emerald water had wide sidewalks that called to my runner's instincts. So Terri and I went for a run. We frequently ran together, especially on weekends and vacations. Normally, I'd have chosen to run across the bridge, continue to the ocean, and keep going for some time along the palm-lined park that parallels the beach. This time I couldn't keep up with Terri, however, so I veered off to a less inviting path along a golf course. I pushed myself stubbornly despite resistance from my legs. After slowing to a jog, my knees buckled and I nearly collapsed. I stumbled over to the nearest palm tree and leaned against it for several minutes. Finally, I decided to walk back to the house. By then I was worried.

When Jessica and I used to take walks back home, I'd instigate our "excuse me" game as we called it. I'd walk in front of her bumping her off the sidewalk and into the bushes and then she'd return me the favor. Now, on our last day of our holiday, as we walked from the ocean beach to the cottage where we were staying, Jessica instigated our little game with a gentle push. To her surprise and Terri's I fell sideways onto the grass like a poorly rooted scarecrow. Terri and Jessica helped me up, stunned and a little amused at my apparent helplessness.

When I got back home I went to see my doctor, Jeffrey Sherman. He sent me to Perry Richardson, a neurologist at George Washington University. The fingers in both my hands were starting to buzz and stiffen, making it difficult to write or type. My legs were now continuing to weaken, and just walking was becoming difficult. Dr. Richardson performed various exams and ordered an MRI.

"I can see nothing the matter with you," he said. "Except, perhaps, for this slightly bulging disc." He pointed to a shadow on the MRI. Dr. Richardson's specialty is neuromuscular disease. My muscles were fine, he said.

With each visit he seemed more and more skeptical of my insistence that something was wrong. Could I be making it all up? No way. I don't have a rich enough fantasy life. This all has to be real. But what's going on and why? Am I the next big medical mystery? I know I shouldn't think this way, but why me? Why now? Just as I'm on the top of my game my body is starting to betray me.

Throughout January my symptoms gradually grew more pronounced. The weakness in my limbs, the buzzing in my hands and feet, told me something was very wrong. This much I knew. But the progression was too slow to give the doctors a clue. Fortunately, because I was a lawyer, I could continue with my work. If I had been a forest ranger or a soccer coach who relied on strength and agility to perform his job, I'd really have been in trouble. As it was, my caseload kept me sufficiently occupied so I couldn't dwell on my physical ailments all day.

Dr. Richardson puzzled over me for six agonizing weeks before he and the chief neurologist, John Kelly, diagnosed me with CIDP, an immune mediated neuropathy. I'd learn more about this bizarre illness in the time ahead. For now, I knew only that my immune system was attacking my peripheral nerves, and so my muscles weren't receiving the necessary signals. The good news was that I could get better soon with treatment. What a relief, to know what was wrong with me and that I'd get better. It was February and with luck I'd be running around the Tidal Basin again by spring.

The doctors prescribed immunosuppressant therapy, consisting of prednisone and IV infusions. But in the weeks ahead my gait grew weaker rather than stronger. Terri, who had been in a state of denial that anything major could be wrong, now realized this was no small thing. She bought me a straight cane to help me up curbs and steps. I enrolled in physical therapy one day a week at the George Washington Medical Center. Using my cane, I walked the mile from my downtown office to GW, a route that took me past Lafayette Park and up Pennsylvania Avenue to the university area in Foggy Bottom. That worked okay for a few weeks, but one day in early March, I collapsed in front of the White House. A man and a woman rushed over to help me to my feet. Embarrassed, I thanked them and continued on my way. The therapists instructed me to buy a four- pronged cane for greater support.

My walking became unsteady, almost tipsy, as if I'd just downed a pitcher of margaritas. My friends and office colleagues were stunned. I stayed at my desk as much as possible to avoid questions. But I couldn't hole up in my office all day long. A paralegal I worked with on occasion stopped me in the hallway by the mailboxes. "What's wrong, Michael? Your walking is funny. " I tried to explain my condition to her as best I could.

Other colleagues gathered around. "He's been diagnosed with some kind of neuropathy," someone said, sparing me the need to repeat myself.

My hopes for a quick recovery transformed gradually into disappointment and then despair. I complained to my doctors and asked for more medicine and more therapy. But nothing they did seemed to help. Terri and I bought a three-wheel rolling walker so I could maintain a level of mobility. In a matter of weeks I'd gone from using a straight cane, to a four-pronged cane, to a rolling walker. What's next, a wheelchair? I kept this thought to myself, but I felt squeamish and frightened, a backcountry explorer being swallowed by quicksand.

Since I could no longer run, my options for continuing to exercise had become limited. Although I had never been a gym rat, Terri insisted that we join a fitness center near our home so that at least I could swim. I agreed. One unusually hot Sunday in mid-April, we planned to go to the pool after Terri ran some errands at the neighborhood CVS pharmacy and Safeway. In the meantime, I would go outdoors and read. My memory of this moment remains painful.

I must cross the alley behind our apartment building to reach the adjoining small park. The park is for the use of condo residents only. How many times have I played frisbee with Jessica here or picnicked with neighbors? The alley, the same one where I taught

Jessica to ride a two-wheeler years ago, is gently sloped on either side, and I find the simple task of crossing it scarier than ever.

I struggle with the help of my walker, stopping midway to look about. The dogwoods are starting to bud and the air is thick with pollen. If I cross the park there is a bench with some shade, but I'm afraid that is too far for me right now. I might collapse if I try to traverse the grass to reach that bench and I'll not be able to get up on my own. I'll wind up lying on the grass like a broken tree limb until someone happens by. Instead, I sit down on one of the wooden benches by the alley without shade. I take my book out of the plastic grocery bag hooked onto my walker and start to read. It's a book about the Brooklyn Dodgers by Doris Kerns Goodwin, called "Wait 'til Next Year."

Even though it's only April, it's in the 80's and perspiration rolls down my forehead and dampens my shirt collar. Part of it must be how weak I feel. I think I'll try to walk over to the bench that has shade, only I'm having trouble lifting myself up. Try again: one, two three, up. On second thought, I'd better stay put for now.

After a couple of hours, Jessica and her boyfriend, Daniel, happen by. I try to get up to greet them but I can't budge. I put both hands on the bench and try again, willing myself up with all my might, but I have no might. This isn't happening. How can I be so weak? Nothing the doctors have done is helping or curing me. As if pushed out of an airplane without a parachute, I keep on falling.

Jessica rushes over and helps me up. Trying to stand, I'm now sweating as if I'd emerged from a steam bath. Daniel stays with me as Jessica goes upstairs to see if Terri has returned from her errands. The two of them soon appear and scamper over to where I sit. Then Jane, my work colleague of many years who lives nearby, shows up. The ladies, Daniel, and I embark on what should be an uneventful trip to our apartment house and back upstairs. Only now, I can't take a step without collapsing to the pavement.

"Are we taking him to GW?" Jane asks Terri, who has just appeared.

"Yes, right now. I'll get the car. Then we'll go upstairs and alert his doctor. Daniel, you wait here with Michael." Terri, usually so

calm and upbeat, is frantic.

Daniel helps me make it the few feet to the side of the building while Terri drives the car around. With a sense of profound relief, I accede to their urging to immediately check into GW Hospital.

By now, I can no longer walk.

3 CIDP

I had arrived at the GW campus early that morning back in February when first I learned of my diagnosis and could still walk. Instead of going right to my appointment, I sat down on a bench in the quadrangle behind the law school library where, decades earlier, I had spent many a day studying my law books or hanging out before class. On this morning, I'd passed the time by watching law students and college kids, some shouldering back packs, others clutching Starbucks coffee in mittened hands, hurrying to and from their classes. So young and spry.

When it got close to the hour of my appointment, I headed back up 22nd street to the old orange brick medical building and took the elevator to the neurology department on the seventh floor. I signed in and was shown to the technician in charge of administering the electro diagnostic testing. She introduced herself as Mary. This was my second experience with these tests, so I knew the drill. I took off my clothes, put on the hospital gown left for me, and lay down on my back on the narrow cot next to the wall, my eyes glued to the murals of faraway seaside retreats plastered on the ceiling. In the meantime, Mary apologetically commenced to prick and shock me for what seemed like the longest half hour in human history.

As I lay there, I thought back on the several weeks since early January when I'd returned home with my family from Vero Beach, after nearly collapsing while jogging. These last few weeks had been a frightening time, a bad dream from which I couldn't wake.

Upon our arrival back in Washington, I had immediately sought medical help. I wanted desperately to figure out what was wrong with me. Not knowing was the worst part. I went alone on my visits to Dr. Richardson who, at first, seemed skeptical of my complaints. Perry Richardson was anything but your cozy Dr. Welby type. A boyish looking forty something, he dressed preppie and spoke in medical terms, guided strictly by the book: "the medical evidence suggests that" or "we now believe such and such to be the case." No warm and fuzzy bedside manner from him. Nevertheless, he was, according to *Washingtonian Magazine*, one of the leading experts in neuromuscular disease in the D.C. area. I was glad to be under his care. I didn't need personality, I wanted answers.

He had me walk in a straight line and tested my muscles and sensory capabilities by administering standard neurologic exams. All of my weaknesses and deficiencies—the tingling in my hands, the numbness in my feet—seemed to be bilateral, impacting my left and right arms and legs the same way. No known neuromuscular disease explained this. He scratched his head. He sent me off for my first set of electromagnetic and nerve conduction tests. For 45 minutes needles pricked my limbs producing mini electro shocks. To hell with the discomfort; I just needed to know what on earth was wrong with me. But the results of these tests yielded no clue.

At the office, Jane combed through *Merck's Manual*, a well-known guide to medical ailments. She guessed multiple sclerosis. Another colleague suggested Lou Gehrig's disease. Were they making bets? "No," I said. "Dr. Richardson has confidently ruled these out." I was trying to reassure myself as much as them.

Finally, in late February, Dr. Richardson sat me down after one of his routine examinations. "I've got a hunch," he said. "I think you have a peripheral neuropathy of some kind." To test his hypothesis, he had arranged for me to take this second series of EMG /nerve conduction tests. Now, with the tests about to be completed, Dr. Richardson's hunch might be validated. I was anxious to find out and I didn't have to wait long for the results.

Dr. Richardson came into the cubicle and greeted me warmly, a rare display for him. "How are you today, partner?" We shook hands.

"Seems I'm still getting worse. My foot balance is way off. The buzzing sensation now affects the whole of my hands and feet. I sure hope you can figure this out today."

"Well, we'll soon see. I'm just going to take a look at the graphs, and then we'll talk. In the meantime you can put your clothes back on."

After studying the graphs generated by the testing, he ushered me into his office. He seemed unusually upbeat. He showed none of the skepticism he'd displayed during my early visits. I, however, was on pins and needles. Was he about to solve the mystery? I was a defendant in criminal court, standing on the edge of an abyss, waiting for the jury to return with its verdict, a verdict that would surely impact the rest of my life.

"Just as I thought," Dr. Richardson said. "These results, when we look at them in concert with the testing we did about a month ago, suggest a diagnosis of Chronic Inflammatory Demyelinating Polyneuropathy." He was confident. "Dr. Kelly has taken a look and he concurs."

Dr. Richardson went on to explain that my condition, commonly referred to as CIDP, is believed to be an immune mediated neuropathy. "You can clearly see the demyelination." I peered over his shoulder at the section of the graphs to which he was pointing. I might as well have been looking at hieroglyphics.

He explained that this type of neuropathy is slow to come on, hence it is considered chronic rather than acute. The acute counterpart of this condition is called Guillain-Barre syndrome, which acts fast, sometimes paralyzing patients within a day or two. I knew about Guillain-Barre from my work on toxic tort cases. I recalled claims in one case that Guillain-Barre syndrome was caused by a toxic exposure of some sort. I didn't think those allegations had been proven, but I did know that Guillain-Barre had been medically linked to certain inoculations, such as those given for typhoid. I'd received inoculations like these when I'd journeyed to Africa.

Dr. Richardson explained that, unlike Guillain-Barre, CIDP is idiopathic. I was intimately familiar with this medical term. An expert witness of mine, a toxicologist, once testified in court, "I like to think of it this way: idiopathic means the doctor's an idiot, he doesn't know the cause." In other words there was no known cause for CIDP. "We believe that the disease is immune mediated," Dr. Richardson repeated. "But we don't yet know what triggers the immune system to behave that way."

I listened intently as Dr. Richardson went on. He explained generally that the nervous system consists of two parts. The Central Nervous System (CNS) is made up of the brain and the spinal cord, while the Peripheral Nervous System (PNS) is made up of a network of nerves that come out from the CNS to other parts of the body. The nerves in the PNS have insulation called myelin sheath that is needed for smooth transmission of nerve impulses or messages. According to prevailing theory, in CIDP a virus or some sort of infection activates the immune system into high gear, but when the virus or infection has been licked, the immune system does not shut down as it is supposed to do. There is something about the myelin sheath, the insulation around the nerves, that mimics the virus or infection. So the antibodies that fought off the virus continue to attack the peripheral nerves. "The good news," he continued, "is that once the immune system is suppressed, damage to the myelin tends to heal quickly, much more quickly than if there is nerve (or axon) damage." I started to feel somewhat relieved.

"And there is an established protocol for treatment. I am going to ask Dr. Kelly to explain a little more about how the disease process works and to go over the treatment protocol." Dr. Richardson left briefly in order to summon Dr. Kelly whose office was just down the hall. My stomach did a back flip as I waited for news about my treatment.

John Kelly was the chief neurologist at GW, and the one possessing the greatest expertise in neuropathy. In his late forties, or early fifties, with receding red hair, Dr. Kelly is a man of few words. He came into the office and got right to the point.

"Generally, we have experienced a great deal of success with two types of treatment used in concert," he said. "We will start you on prednisone, which is a steroid used to suppress the inflammation around the myelin. Next, we administer what is referred to as intravenous immunoglobulin, which we refer to in shorthand as IVIgG."

He explained the way IVIgG works. By flooding the body with the good antibodies such as IgG, the immune system is altered. IVIgG is administered as an infusion into the vein and is less invasive than other treatments. The therapy should be repeated every three to four weeks for as long as necessary. "We'll admit you into the hospital this weekend for a first round," Dr. Kelly said. "For subsequent treatments we can arrange for it to be done at home."

"This is all good news, of course," he added, almost as an afterthought. "There is no bad news."

A huge sense of relief flooded through me, a calming sea after a bad storm. "How long will it take for me to start to get better?" I asked.

"Not long since myelin has the capacity to regenerate quickly. Some patients start to feel better within a matter of days after the first IVIgG."

Dr. Richardson's nurse made the arrangements for my upcoming treatment at the hospital, and then I thanked everyone and left. A monumental weight had just been lifted from my shoulders.

As I walked back to DuPont Circle, my step was lighter than when I had made the trip earlier that morning. I heard myself humming old show tunes. I'll feel some improvement after this weekend. Can't wait to tell everyone. This will turn out to be just a bump in the road, after all. By April, I'll be able, once again, to run around the tidal basin during lunch break, gazing at the cherry blossoms while dodging tourists. On weekends, I'll jog into the park, weaving under the dogwoods in their pink and white regalia. Tonight, we'll celebrate. Tomorrow I'll tell the world. What I didn't realize right then was that in the days and weeks ahead,

Terri and I would discover additional information about CIDP, not all of it as rosy and bright as the picture painted by Drs. Kelly and Richardson.

When I got home I phoned Terri with the news. "Thank God," she said. "What a relief just to know what's going on and that you can be fixed." Then I phoned Dr. Sherman, my internist.

"You turned out to be interesting," he said. "Not something as simple as we had hoped, but interesting."

"Both Dr. Kelly and Dr. Richardson said the prognosis for full recovery is good," I insisted. "I should begin to see progress as early as next week, after my treatment."

"I just don't want you to set your hopes too high." His voice was gentle, but matter of fact. "Nobody can truly predict the outcome with something like this. The treatments work for some people, but there remains much to learn in this area and, for the present, it's still a lot like voodoo medicine."

I thanked him, but as I hung up my heart sank to my feet. He sure has a different take on this, I thought. Terri's Uncle Howard, also a doctor who had suffered from a rare neurologic condition, said much the same thing as Dr. Sherman. "Everyone is different," said Howard. "No one, including your doctors, really knows what to expect. Whatever you do, stay clear of the Internet or you'll drive yourself loony."

I thanked him for his thoughts and hung up. Now, the high I was feeling on the way home came crashing down like the blade of a guillotine. My brain was in turmoil. I poured myself a glass of wine.

What if the neurologists are wrong? What if the treatments don't work? What if I keep getting worse?

No, stop this nonsense. You haven't even had the first treatment yet. Prednisone is a miracle drug, they say.

But who are they? This is no sure thing and it's foolish to pretend so. It's unpredictable. Unpredictable. Unpredictable. Unpredictable.

Come on you, stop this right now. You have to keep your head.

But how should I think? Whom should I trust? My own body is betraying me.

I drank a second glass of wine, and then a third.

In the days following my first IVIgG treatment in the hospital, I anxiously awaited signs of improvement. At some point I was supposed to reduce my prednisone dosage to every other day. I protested to Dr. Richardson's nurse, Barbara, that I wasn't seeing improvement, that I needed more, not less, prednisone. "My goodness, you just had IVIgG last week. You must give it time," she said. She must think I'm one big complainer.

Terri went on line to search for as much information about CIDP as she could find. Jane sought out *Merck's Manual* and other medical treatises on hand in the Torts Branch library. I was very much a textbook case. One treatise described the first symptoms of CIDP as consisting of tingling, prickling, burning, and sensory loss in the balls of the feet and tips of the toes. That was me to a tee. In the section headed "Recovery From Neuropathy" it noted that peripheral nerve fibers have an excellent ability to regenerate *under proper circumstances*. What could that mean, I wondered. What are proper circumstances?

I read on. What I discovered was that whether regeneration took place depended on whether the cause of the neuropathy had been eliminated. This meant that the treatments had better work for me or else. Also, while patients with demylenation but no secondary axonal degeneration (in other words, the nerves, themselves, were intact) could fully recover from paralysis to normal strength within three to four weeks, axonal regeneration could take from two months to more than a year, depending on the severity of the neuropathy and the length of regeneration required. What this meant to me was that the longer the treatments didn't work, the greater the chance that I'd suffer axonal, or real nerve damage, making recovery slow and uncertain.

The more I read the more concerned I became. The treatment protocols chosen for me seemed reasonable, but less clear were the response rates for the different treatments. Against her uncle's advice, Terri found a chat room for CIDP patients and discovered that there were a wide variety of outcomes and responses to the types of treatments I was receiving.

As the weeks slogged by and I started to feel worse rather than better, my concern turned to anxiety, and before long anxiety turned to desperation. By mid-March, I called Dr. Richardson's office to schedule a second IVIgG treatment, and it seemed they took forever to respond. When the nurse came to my apartment to administer the infusion, I pumped her for information on the chances for success. I grasped at anything, any basis for optimism. All she could say was it depends on the individual. Not what I hoped to hear.

After it appeared to me that I wasn't responding to the second IVIgG, Jane suggested I get a second opinion, perhaps at Johns Hopkins in Baltimore. I hesitated. "My doctors are the best in the area," I said. It just seemed like an arduous process. But, around the time of my third IVIgG in April, Jane emailed a neurologist, Dr. Jim Albers, who practiced in the Mid-West and who had served as an expert witness for me in a Jacksonville, Florida case some years before. In researching CIDP, Jane had noticed that in 1998 Dr. Albers had commented on a paper about CIDP. She mentioned in her email that I was under the care of Dr. Richardson at GW and had seen Dr. Kelly once on consult. She asked whether he could recommend someone, possibly at Hopkins, who could provide a second opinion.

Dr. Albers replied to Jane's message within days. He said that he and Dr. Kelly were good friends having trained together at the Mayo Clinic. He noted that Dr. Kelly was recognized for his clinical research in CIDP. Dr. Albers gave the names of doctors at Hopkins that I could see for a second opinion if I wanted, but also said that he didn't think that they had any greater clinical experience than Dr. Kelly.

Dr. Albers added that the good news was that 85 percent of CIDP patients responded to suppression of the immune system, although it could take weeks to plateau and most patients require long-term treatment. He wished me well.

I was happy to receive the response from Dr. Albers and grateful that Jane had undertaken the communication. I think Terri, Jane and I were all persuaded that a second opinion was unnecessary so long as Dr. Kelly remained on my case as a consult.

I was confident that he would.

But by this time I had already checked into GW Hospital. I was a quadriplegic.

4 Terri's Mountain

On that April day when I couldn't walk anymore, when I'd take one or two steps with my walker before collapsing to my knees, my family, together with our friend Jane, decided to check me into the hospital. Daniel waited with me as I leaned against the car by the little park behind our apartment house, while Terri and Jessica went upstairs with Jane. It was then, I later learned, in the living room of our apartment, well out of my sight, that the dam burst for my wife and daughter, all of their pent up worries and frustration giving way to a torrent of tears, an outpouring of their unspoken fears. Jane, our loyal friend, our rock, took control of the moment. First, she reassured Terri and Jessica. Then she called the hospital to make sure that the senior neurologist on duty would expect me. My wife and daughter collected themselves and came downstairs with Jane. Together, we sped to the emergency room.

By this point, Terri had come to realize that physically I was no longer the person she'd married. Over a few months, I had been transformed from an active, vibrant middle-aged man into someone who would require care and assistance in virtually every facet of daily life. Perhaps that is why she, like me, had been in denial about the potential seriousness of my condition. At some point the treatments would surely kick in, we told each other, and I'd magically revert to the way I used to be. Who were we kidding?

Terri and I had met in February 1997, two days after I turned 50, and just two and a half years before the onset of my illness. We were both trial lawyers at the Justice Department, she with the Office of Immigration Litigation, and I with the office of Environmental Torts. We did not meet through work, however. Both of us were into running and were introduced by a mutual friend, Bridgid, who had worked first in my office and then in Terri's. Terri hosted a party at her townhouse in Maryland the evening following a 10K road race. I almost didn't go. I'd felt drowsy and lay down on the sofa around the time I needed to leave. I figured I'd just skip this one party, but Jessica, then 15, would have none of it. I'd been divorced from her mom for nearly ten years, and a single dad for eight years following her mom's death. "Dad," she said, "go to the party, you might meet somebody. You won't meet anyone staying here watching TV." And so, I drove from our Connecticut Avenue condo into the Maryland suburbs to party and socialize.

Terri was short with olive skin, a mass of dark, curly hair, and bore a wide, bright smile. She was smart, effervescent, and 16 years my junior. Plus, she looked really cute in her blue corduroy jump suit. We chatted. I told her she seemed young to have her own house. She laughed. "I'm not that young," she said. A week later I asked her out to dinner at my favorite Thai restaurant in Cleveland Park.

We hit it off immediately, although that might not have been the case had we met a year or so sooner. "I used to chain smoke and eat junk food. I dated the wrong guys for all the wrong reasons," she said. "Then, this past year, my house mate and I joined a gym and started running. Now, I'm in better shape than I was in my twenties. I mean, maybe that's not saying much. But, it's true. I was a total sloth back then."

"What about the smoking?"

"Oh, I've quit completely," she fibbed. As she confessed to me later, she was in the process of quitting, but she knew I was a runner and didn't want me to think that she still smoked, even a little. During smoking breaks at work she'd wander several blocks from her office so none of my colleagues at Torts would catch her smoking. In time she'd come to realize this charade was ridiculous, so she willed herself to quit altogether.

Ignoring the advice from friends that you never talk about your divorce during a first date, I told her the long, sorrowful story of my marriage to Jessica's mom, and its impact on Jessica. "I was living in a war zone," I said, "and didn't realize soon enough that it was better to leave than not."

"That sounds just like my folks," she said. "My mom and dad were at each other's throats while I was in high school. Ashtrays and china bowls would fly across the room. They've been divorced more than a decade now and my mom refuses to put it behind her."

We discovered that we both came from Jewish backgrounds, although neither of us was very religious. Terri had grown up in the Squirrel Hill neighborhood of Pittsburgh, while I was a New York City boy. I explained how my remaining New York family—my cousins, Patsy and Judy, and Aunt Ceal—would be relieved if I found a "nice Jewish girl," especially in light of my disastrous first marriage. "They've even threatened to screen the women I date," I said. "Jessica considers herself Episcopalian, like her mom. So I call her an episca-yiddle." I explained that Jessica was learning disabled and had trouble with abstract thinking. "When she was eight I told her she was half Jewish. She asked which half, top or bottom."

Terri and I felt comfortable with each other and our relationship took off like a shuttle hurled into space. On our second date we went to an old *Star Trek* movie at the *Uptown* on Connecticut Avenue. Timid at first, I moved my hand slowly toward hers, and sensing my shyness, she reached for mine. The ice broken, we smooched shamelessly throughout the film. When it was over, we staggered out of the theater and crossed the street for a dinner of pizza and wine.

My shyness wasn't a new thing for me. I was a late bloomer when it came to dating. In high school, nailing a date for the annual prom was my nemesis. I went to a small private school on Manhattan's east side, across the park from where I lived with my extended family. You didn't go to the prom if you didn't have a date. I despised the girls in my class, or maybe feared them is more like it. If prom time came and I didn't have a date, the dreaded social committee (consisting of all girls, of course) would be sure to get one for me, whether I wanted one or not, a happenstance I didn't relish. I imagined Andrea with her green eyes and pink glasses—or was it pink eyes and green glasses—smiling as she informed me she'd found me a date, an offer I dare not refuse.

But junior year I outsmarted them, or so I thought. I got a date with a girl named Jan I'd met at a softball game in Central Park—two months before the prom. She seemed nice, not all stuck up like the girls in my class. We chatted, I asked her to the prom, she accepted. Well that's a monkey off my back, I figured. My only dilemma: what to do in the meantime. I didn't have a clue.

I recall the following conversation at dinnertime less than a week before the prom:

"Dinner is served, everybody come to the table," my grandmother announces.

I take my usual place at the table. "What about Sis and Lou?" I ask. "Aren't we waiting for them?"

"Your mother's working late again," Aunt Ceal says. "Goodness knows where Lou is."

"Patsyee, Juuudyee, dinnnerrr," Ceal calls down the hall for my cousins to hop to it.

My grandparents who we called Mom and Pop take their places at one end with Ceal and the girls opposite me.

"What's for dinner?" Judy, my oldest cousin, is short with dark curly hair and dark brown skin, a tribute to years of sun worshipping.

"Meatloaf and mashed potatoes," Mom says.

"Again? We just had that the other day."

"Last Friday," Mom says indignantly.

"This is Tuesday," Pop snarls.

"Hey Jude," Patsy turns to her sister. "How was your date Saturday? I took a little glimpse while the two of you were walking out. He was the spitting image of Howdy Doody." They both laugh hilariously. Patsy is exactly one year older than me. She's much

taller than her sister with light brown hair and lily-white skin. Both girls, though very different from one another, are attractive and popular.

"Awful," Judy says. "Did you notice the yellow leisure suit he was wearing? What a jerk. I had the absolute worst time ever. He barely spoke at all, just picked at his zits all night long. A real loser."

Ceal joins in the laughter, as she puts out one Chesterfield and lights another.

"Mikey," Patsy turns to me grinning. "Do you have a date for the prom yet? Saturday's coming up, you know."

"Don't call me that and yes, I have a date. So there."

"Since when? Judy asks.

"About two and a half months ago when I asked her."

"Oh my God, mommy, did you hear that," Patsy cries out hollering hysterically as she grabs her mother's arm. Judy, so taken up with the hilarity of the moment, coughs up her food. Ceal too laughs out loud, her eyes now watering. Mom and Pop are in their own world. Pop says something to Mom in Hungarian, the language of the old country that they use sparingly, when they don't want us youngsters to understand.

I suddenly have a vision. I imagine Patsy's hairdo enhanced with fistfuls of meatloaf and potatoes from my plate.

"How does she know you're still coming?" Judy asks. Still giggling. "Don't you think you should call her?"

"Of course I'll call her. This week. I'll let her know to meet me at the subway near her apartment."

"Oh my God, Judy. Did you hear that?" Patsy again bursts into a fit of hysteria. "The subway!" Maybe she'll have a convulsion and die, I think. Maybe they all will.

"Michael, really," Ceal says. "This is the prom. What's she gonna do, wait on the street in her gown? Take a taxi. Sis will give you the money if you need it. And you really should call her."

I get up from the table, un-excused, and head over to my mother's room where there's a telephone and I can speak privately. I shut the door and dial Jan's number. I hold my breath.

"Hello." It's a girl's voice. Maybe it's Jan. Can't be sure.

"Hello, is Jan home?"

"I'm Jan. Who is this?"

"This is Michael, remember. We're going to the prom this Saturday. I thought I'd pick you up in a taxi around seven. Is that good for you?" Silence. A long, painful silence.

"Michael? Oh, Michael. Of course. Michael, I'm awfully sorry but it's been so long since we spoke. I thought for sure you forgot and so I've got other plans for this Saturday night. I'm so sorry, but I expected you'd call much sooner. I'm really, really sorry."

I swallowed hard. "Oh that's okay, I understand." More silence.

"Well I guess I'll see you at the game the next time we play you," is all I can think to say.

"Sure, I'll see you then."

I slink back to the dining room table ever so quietly. Maybe no one will notice me.

"Well," Judy asks.

"Well what?"

"Do you still have a date?"

"Of course."

What happened afterward is fuzzy, but no doubt the Social Committee once again came to my rescue.

By the time I'd met Terri I'd come a long way since high school, but dating had never come easy for me. The antithesis of a womanizer, I lacked self-assurance in asking women out and often bumbled on first dates. My tumultuous first marriage helped mature me, but shyness was part of my DNA. With Terri, however, I felt comfortable and more confident. My initial shyness abated as soon as the ice was broken on that second date when we smooched throughout the *Star Trek* movie. I sensed she was the right woman for me, and our relationship evolved from that point on.

The Saturday following our second date was the day before the Saint Paddy's Day 10K race. Terri came to a carbo-loading party at my apartment that evening and slept over. With her help, I overcame any lingering timidity I might have felt that night.

Within the first month of our budding romance, she accepted

my invitation to spend a spring weekend in New York City with Jessica and me. "You can meet my zany family," I said.

"Not as crazy as mine, I bet." Seems we were in competition.

We took a hotel room on Central Park South while Jessica stayed with my aunt on the Upper West Side. Closed to traffic on weekends, the park in spring is a glorious mosaic of flowers, green lawns, joggers and bikers. We reserved Saturday morning to run the full six-mile loop through the park. We saved the remainder of the day for visits with family.

On Sunday, the three of us rode the subway to lower Manhattan, where we met my childhood friend Arthur and his wife Liz, for brunch. Arthur and Liz had suffered with me through one failed marriage, so I was anxious for them to like Terri. As it turned out, they hit it off with her from the start. Arthur asked her about her work in immigration and Liz joined in, all of them ignoring me. That was fine though, because I knew that Arthur and Liz recognized that this time I'd made a wise choice.

After brunch we all boarded the ferry for a tour of Ellis Island, the entry point for the hundreds of thousands of immigrants seeking refuge in a new land decades ago. Terri had never visited there despite her work in the field of immigration.

Trying to look her best to impress my family and friends, Terri hadn't worn her most comfortable walking shoes. Big mistake. One of my favorite things about my city is walking through the varied neighborhoods, and I was eager to show her my old haunts on foot. So after the tour, we scrambled off the boat, bid good-bye to my friends, and began what my daughter referred to as a forced march.

The year after law school I had clerked for a federal judge with chambers in the United States Courthouse at Foley Square. During those days when it stayed light until seven or eight in the evening, I'd often walk the four miles from work to my basement apartment in a brownstone on West End Avenue, close to where I grew up. Through Chinatown, Little Italy, SoHo, Greenwich Village, and straight up Broadway I'd meander, taking in the sights, sounds, and smells, stopping for a pastry in Little Italy or a takeout meal of kabobs from a food cart in the Village. Now I led Terri and Jessica on a tour of each of these neighborhoods as far north as the Village where we came to rest at a cozy eatery with white tablecloths. Later, I showed mercy to my little troop, hailing a taxi to take us to our respective abodes uptown.

After Jessica and I returned home, I asked her what she thought of Terri. "The two of you were acting ditzy and air-brained," she said. Typical teenager. I couldn't argue with her on that, but I got the feeling she felt comfortable with Terri. In the months ahead, the three of us went on weekend outings together, including sojourns to the beach during summer. Eventually Terri moved in with Jessica and me. At first she stayed over on weekends, but I gave her a key and asked her to bring over some clothes. Before long she was living with us. I thought I'd better break the news to my daughter. "Jessica, Terri will be moving in with us this week."

"DAD," said an incredulous Jessica, "she already has. If you haven't noticed, I have." Clueless dad.

Suddenly, marriage seemed a strong possibility.

Before long I got my chance to meet Terri's folks, separately. Her mom, Eleanor, had once been a professional actress, and the theater remained in her blood. Unfortunately, functioning in the real world wasn't her forte. To be happy, she needed to be the center of attention, a prima donna. She was prone to tantrums if she didn't have her way.

My first introduction to Eleanor came a month or two after our New York trip when we picked her up at the bus terminal in D.C. She was to stay with us for a week. As soon as we helped her unload her bags into the hatch of my Subaru wagon she began to talk non-stop, telling me of Terri's childhood accomplishments and embarrassing moments. Several times I tried to get a word in edgewise but always in vain. This woman has boundary issues, I thought. Some months later when our relationship was on solid footing, Terri confided that she'd worried that her mother would frighten me away as she had many an earlier boyfriend.

My daughter turned out to be the most patient in coping with Eleanor's erratic moods. "Grandma Eleanor," she called her, and they became instant friends. And Eleanor, a part-time schoolteacher in Seattle, was good with kids. She saw to it that Jessica memorized her driver's manual so she could pass the written test and secure a learner's permit.

Terri's dad, Abe, a proud man of Middle-Eastern heritage, seemed happiest when in full control. There was no controlling Eleanor, so it was hard to imagine those two together in an elevator, much less the bedroom. I met Abe for the first time when he came to D.C. one weekend on business several months after Terri and I had been dating. He, Terri and I met for Sunday brunch at a small uptown eatery. "What are your intentions toward my daughter?" was one of the first things he asked me. I wasn't prepared for the third degree, but I think I convinced him my intentions were honorable.

Terri's only sibling, her older sister Lara, also lived in Seattle. Lara was a singer, songwriter, and lawyer, in that order. She couldn't have been more different from Terri. Terri was creative but also pragmatic, content with a stable life style that entailed a fixed paycheck deposited automatically every two weeks, while Lara seemed comfortable riding the waves of one risky enterprise after another.

When I first met Lara I could sense she was evaluating me. Was I too old for her little sister? Was I hip enough? Dining at a bistro not far from my Connecticut apartment, Lara regaled us with tales of her latest music projects. Then she turned to me. "Michael, who's your favorite female vocalist?" I looked straight at her, resisting the urge to smile. "Ethel Merman," I said. I don't think she knew what to make of me.

After a courtship of about six months, Terri and I got engaged, and in May 1998, we were married at the Arts Club of Washington, a small, elegant townhouse boasting a lovely courtyard and within walking distance of the White House. It was no surprise that Eleanor showed up late, missing some of the photo shoot. Before I entered the picture, Terri and her mom were habitually late to appointments or events. Terri told me about the time she and her mom were assigned the task of bringing a cooked turkey to a family dinner one Thanksgiving. They showed up an hour late with an uncooked bird. After that the family would fib about the hour set for a dinner invitation, telling them to come an hour before, and never again asked them to bring the main course.

Now, we looked all around the courtyard, but no Eleanor. Would she throw a fit if we proceeded without her? I could sense Terri's anxiety as she kept a lookout, anticipating her mother's grand entrance. We gave the photographer the green light to begin shooting. The wedding guests were starting to shuffle in, but not Eleanor. I envisioned her arriving hours late, missing the ceremony, fuming that we hadn't waited, and storming out. Luckily, in the end, she arrived in time to pose for a few family photos, so a potential disaster was averted.

Terri's sister brought her rock band across country as part of a planned road trip. Her gift to us was to have her band, which included her boyfriend and future husband, Maurice, play at our wedding. Estranged from her dad, Lara took us aside to announce she was two months pregnant, and swore us to secrecy. Her dad wouldn't understand about her relationship with the bass player in her band, much less her pregnancy by him. But we soon learned that she had made the same pronouncement to half the guests, including family members on her dad's side, swearing each to secrecy.

Abe's two young children by his second marriage, Victor and Alexis, served as ring boy and flower girl. Terri's mom and dad walked her down the aisle and never spoke a word to each other. Our wedding was a delicate balancing act.

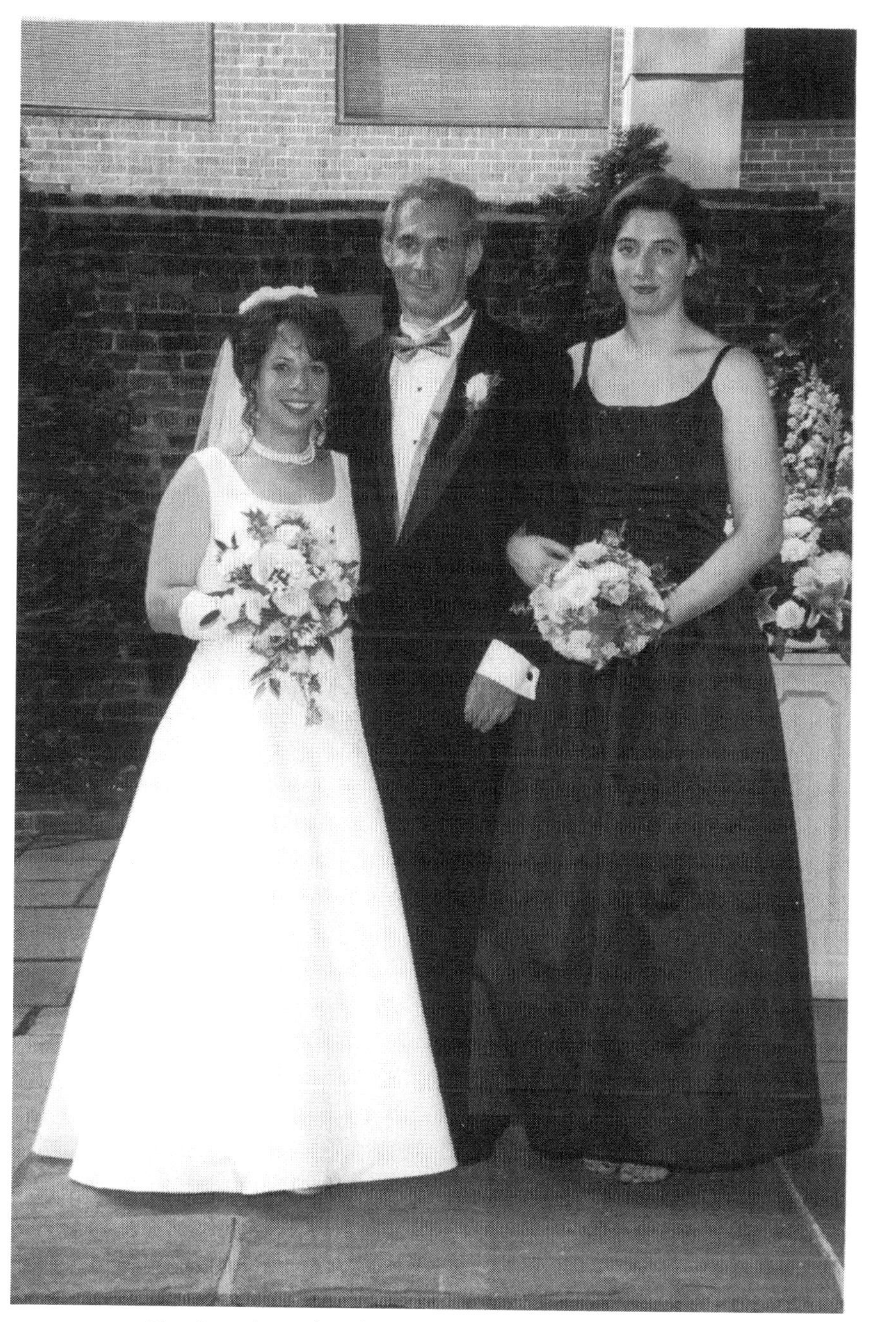

Terri and Michael married at the Arts Club of Washington, May 16, 1998, here with Jessica

On our honeymoon, after spending a few days on our own in Florence and Venice, we walked with British travelers through the hill towns, vineyards, and olive groves of Tuscany. We walked through fields thick with gorse, and picnicked beneath cypress trees, feasting on cheeses, olives, salads made with pears and Gorgonzola, prosciutto, Salami Chingale, breads, fruits and local wines. One day, after picnicking in a barn, we napped on haystacks cradled in each other's arms. At San Gimignano we climbed several of the city's 14 towers at dusk, after the tour buses had left. In Siena, we climbed the bell tower of the Palazzo Publico yielding birds-eye views of the Piazza Del Campo, one of the great open spaces of Europe. Our British companions dubbed us "the wedding couple." "We kept wondering why you'd want to spend your honeymoon with us," one lady quipped. But we were together and happy.

Back home in D.C., we dined at ethnic restaurants, entertained, partied, ran in road races, hiked in the neighboring countryside, listened to jazz and classic rock. In contrast to my tumultuous first marriage in which Jessica's mom and I were constantly at battle, Terri and I became dedicated partners. I introduced her to the wonders of foreign travel, helped her manage her unruly debt, and persuaded her to nurture a healthier, arms-length relationship with her dysfunctional family. She, in turn, helped me navigate the nettlesome teen years of my daughter, and taught me, for the first time, that I could truly love another, something I'd found elusive in my first marriage.

We also complemented each other's strengths and weaknesses. I was the organized one, neat, orderly, timely, a little obsessive-compulsive, and, at times, impatient. Terri was upbeat—"strawberry shortcake" someone once nicknamed her. She loved to cook—mostly comfort foods at first, such as homemade chicken soup that she'd learned from her mom—and loved it even more when I appreciated her cooking. She could be spacey at times ("where did I leave my glasses?"), but praise-be-to-god for my sake, she was patient and good-natured.

Now, as I gradually lost strength and mobility, I gave thanks for my good fortune in having Terri by my side. How could I go through this alone? As I think back on this time, I never doubted she'd support me to the fullest, but I sometimes thought she got a raw deal. What if I didn't recover? Could I expect her to put up with my dependency day in and day out for the rest of time? If she had misgivings, which I now know she had, she didn't let on. If you can't run again, you can at least bike or swim, she'd say. Always looking at the glass half full, not half empty. Strawberry shortcake, indeed. If my illness had happened during my marriage to Sylvia—Jessica's deceased mom—I hear her voice all too well: "get over it, you malingerer." If there was a silver lining in all this, it's that it was happening now and not then.

In the first several weeks after I started noticing something wrong with me, Terri and I separately nurtured a sense of denial that I could be seriously ill. In Terri's mind, after all, I was the one who initiated hiking trips and exotic travel, including our assault on Kilimanjaro. Although she had turned her life around for the better before she met me, in her mind, I was the one who ensured we'd keep to a healthy and vigorous life style. Once a chain smoker, Terri had put cigarettes behind her. The old Terri would have never dreamed of climbing Kilimanjaro. The new Terri couldn't wait to go. The old Terri had battled depression and debt. The new Terri felt more relaxed and confident as we built our lives together. It would turn our world upside down and defy the laws of gravity if I were to become physically dependent on her or anyone else.

The months following our return from our New Year's trip to Vero Beach catapulted us out of our complacency. Together, we embarked on an emotional roller coaster ride. When I returned home from the evidentiary hearing in Texas in mid-February, and my walking seemed worse than ever, Terri said over dinner, "This is no small matter with you. This is turning into a big deal."

At Terri's urging, I started to take long walks since I could no longer jog or run. On weekends in late March and early April, as the daffodils and crocuses burst into bloom, I walked into Rock Creek Park and hobbled along a portion of my former running route. I tried to break into a jog now and then but couldn't do it without risking a fall. As my walking became less steady, I realized that I could no longer climb the steps to the public restrooms in the park without holding onto the stone sidewall. If there were no wall next to the steps, I'd be out of luck. Our roller coaster was now heading down hill and gathering steam.

After my diagnosis in February, when the prescribed treatments failed to heal me, I became less and less stable. One day I could get up from the floor by pushing myself up; the next day I'd need to crawl over to a chair to help me get up. One day I could step up from a curb with the help of my cane; the next day I'd need to find a lower curb or driveway. I would awaken each morning scared that I would find myself weaker than the day before. I often relive the following scene:

It's early morning. Terri is fast asleep, but I need to use the toilet. I hobble to the bathroom with cane in hand. My arms are as weak now as my legs have been for some time. To lift myself off the toilet, I'm now in the habit of pushing hard on the sink next to it. Hopefully, the sink is solid enough to support me. This time it's more difficult than it's been in the past several days. I push with my whole arm and fall forward onto the floor. I can't get up. Terri hears the commotion and runs over to me. After a few unsuccessful tries, she gets me up. "My poor baby." She holds me for a long, long time.

In mid-April, the day before I entered the hospital, Terri and I drove to a warehouse in Virginia in pursuit of a rolling walker. Walking had become a hazard for me resulting in numerous scrapes and bruises on my elbows and knees. The salesman, a burly fellow with a full beard, serenaded us with a pitch about how a wheelchair would afford greater mobility and, hence, independence. "This chair will make you mobile, and then you'll be free to go anywhere without fear."

Terri wanted to shout him down and tell him that he didn't know me. Instead, she felt her eyes well up with tears. She turned her back on us pretending to be intensely interested in the array of mobility aids on display. She didn't want me to see her crying and didn't turn around to face me until her eyes were dry again and she could trust her voice not to falter.

If Terri and I had been in denial about my downhill slide, Jessica wasn't. As I think back on this time, I wish I had been better attuned to the impact my illness was having on her. I would come to know this later, but not yet. I was too busy willing my illness to go away and figuring how to cope when it didn't.

5 Learning to Cope

The drive to George Washington Hospital is filled with adventure—hundreds of young protesters line the streets venting their anger at The International Monetary Fund and World Bank policy meetings now taking place in D.C., but their aims elude me. When I marched against the Vietnam War, my mission seemed clear. I knew what my goals were. I'm not sure what these folks want.

At a police barricade we plead with an officer to allow us through so we can reach the ER without traveling a good distance out of the way. I'm oddly relaxed. I feel the urgency of the moment, but it's coupled with a sense of relief. Managing to get through each day has become a nightmare. Now I can surrender control to others. I don't have to fret over how to handle Passover dinner this week at the home of Terri's aunt and uncle where I'd be the center of attention, everyone watching my wife serve me and cater to me, not to mention feeling sorry for me.

And what about getting around at the office? Having to use my walker just to navigate the way from my desk to the printer or copying machine while carrying case files. How would I manage that trick? How embarrassing to ask my colleagues to help me with such basic tasks. Terri leans over to me. "Your doctors better come up with a new bag of tricks," she says.

"Yes," I say. "Nothing they've tried so far has worked a damn." In the driveway at the ER, I gladly let Terri and Jane take care of

the logistics. I don't want to have to deal, just let the docs and nurses come up with new treatments that will fix me.

My first day at GW was a blur of interviews with administrators, medical interns, residents, doctors, and rides on cots through harshly lit corridors to separate wards for CAT scans and x-rays. Other patients, some with IVs and a maze of tubes, some with oxygen masks, were also pushed along to unknown destinations. If I closed my eyes against these images, I could imagine I was exploring an underwater world amidst snorkelers and scuba divers breathing through tubes and tanks. Certain images remain with me. An obese middle-aged man in a blue and white gown that didn't fit him being rushed along wheezing and coughing through an oxygen mask. A teen-aged boy with his head heavily bandaged sitting up in a wheel chair waiting for god knows what.

If I'd previously felt I wasn't getting enough attention from the doctors, the situation had changed. The four senior neurologists on staff were now following my case closely. I guess I turned out to be interesting, as Dr. Sherman had said.

Dr. Richardson, my treating neurologist and one of The Big Four, was on duty the second day. He strolled into my room followed closely by ten or so medical students or interns. They hovered around him just inside the door to my room. I've long understood that teaching hospitals, like GW, are the best place to be, especially if, like me, you are suffering a rare type of illness. They can also be exhausting, with a steady parade of interns studying patients like props in a classroom.

Dr. Richardson greeted me. He said that he was sorry that my most recent IVIgG treatment the previous week wouldn't have a sufficient chance to work. But he understood my desperation and desire to explore other treatments. "Your neuropathy began slowly, insidiously," he said. "And by now it has really defined itself."

Defined me, he means. I pondered that. Everything had been good, too good perhaps. Marriage, travels to exotic lands, running every day, climbing Kilimanjaro. Suddenly, wham! I'm a helpless cripple dependent on others for everything.

"You might say so," I said to him. I was disappointed and miffed, perhaps unreasonably, that he and Dr. Kelly had been unable to prevent my condition from worsening to this point. Their initial optimism had raised my hopes. But the treatments hadn't worked so far. What if nothing works? What then? I sure can't stay this way.

If I were a true believer I could turn to prayer, but I've never been one, forever the skeptic. Logic is the crutch that's carried me through each day, commonsense my failsafe. But where is the sense to what's happening to me now?

As one of GW's senior neurologists, Dr. Richardson spent much of his time teaching medical students in addition to seeing patients. With ten or more budding doctors listening to him like a guru, he was now in his element.

"Mr. Scadron has been diagnosed with idiopathic CIDP—chronic inflammatory demyelinating polyneuropathy—which we believe is an immune mediated condition affecting the peripheral nervous system. One way of discerning this is the symmetrical nature of symptoms. The limbs on either side of the body are affected in much the same way. Look at the indenture in his hands, for example." He lifted my right hand for the students to see. The muscle wasting below the thumb was easy to detect. He then proceeded to give me his standard neurological exam. He lifted my left arm. "Push my arm," he commanded. I couldn't get his arm to budge any more than if it were a steel pole. "Now resist me," he instructed, as my arm readily gave way to his push. He rated my muscles in each of my arms and legs from one to five, five being relatively normal. Only my shoulders were anywhere close to five. He used pins to test the sense of feeling in my limbs. "Close your eyes. Now tell me if you feel sharp or dull." The bottoms of my feet were so numb, I could hardly feel the bed sheets.

After he had completed his exam and the interns had shuffled out, Dr. Richardson stayed a minute or two to reaffirm the treatment protocol. They would try a series of treatments called plasmapheresis, where blood is drawn and a machine separates out the plasma. The blood is then returned along with artificial plasma consisting of albumin and saline. If I still showed no improvement, they would start me on a six month regimen of Cytoxan—a form of chemotherapy to be performed monthly over a six month period—a smaller dosage than that normally given to cancer patients. It would be administered to me for the purpose of suppressing my hyperactive immune system. He showed me the write-up of one study of a group of 15 patients with CIDP treated with Cytoxan, which indicated that within six months after treatment was initiated, a majority of patients began showing some improvement.

As a lawyer, I was used to working with experts in epidemiology in connection with environmental tort cases. I noted there were only 15 patients in the group, not a truly scientific study. Also, not all of the 15 patients had improved. And six months seemed like an eternity. Bile rose from my gut to my throat at the prospect of being so helpless for so long, with no certainty of getting better.

"Six months is a long time," I complained. I was desperate for some reason to believe—just an ounce of hope—this couldn't be really happening to me, that my condition could be fixed right away, and that my life would be returned to me pronto.

"We had hoped for a quicker response with the prednisone and IVIgG treatment, but the prognosis is still good," Dr. Richardson said. "You are very early into this. Where there is damage only to the myelin surrounding the nerves, recovery can be rapid, but with mixed nerve and myelin damage like you have, it takes a while for the nerves to regenerate and reconnect with the muscles. Where CIDP patients have gotten better, they usually do so in the first year."

If only I could get a nerve transplant, I mused. But I knew there was no such thing. Not for my condition, anyway.

"Generally, the muscles are extremely welcoming," the doctor explained. "But only to a point. After about 18 months, if there is no muscle activity, they won't recognize the nerves and wasting will occur. You should start to feel strength in your upper arms first, as those nerves have a shorter distance to travel. But in 18 months, I would say, you'll pretty much know where you will be long term."

Eighteen months. I'm in a race against time.

When the doctors had left, I glanced at the mirror above the bureau. I could hardly recognize myself now, a shriveled up old codger in a skimpy hospital gown. That sure is a strange man staring back at me. What's he doing here?

Get used to me, he said. I'm here to stay.

As I think back on that time, what I was most afraid of was the need to re-learn my way in the world in order to maintain some semblance of autonomy. I'd never had to struggle so hard for such basic things.

I came of age among an extended family of eight, and we lived in an 11-room apartment on Manhattan's upper west side. My father died before I was born. Patsy likes to recall that he keeled over from a heart attack the day he learned my mother was pregnant. We called my mother Sis because when my older cousin, Judy, was a baby, she couldn't pronounce my mother's given name, Frances. My mother contemplated an abortion, but lucky for me, Uncle Lou said "don't be silly Fran, come live with us." "Us" meant Lou, Patsy, Judy, Aunt Ceal, and our maternal grandparents, Mom and Pop.

As small fry, my cousins and I had nurses and nannies. For as long as I remember, my family employed a cook and a maid. Us kids were all sent to a small private school on the west side that moved to the east side my sophomore year in high school. So I guess you can say we had money. But, unlike the rest of my family, I was always a bit shy about that.

Lou owned an electronics business in Brooklyn that employed up to 100 workers in its heyday. Sis ran the office. The business would eventually fail but while it was healthy, Uncle Lou was generous to us kids with his money, if not his time or praise. He and my mother put me through college and law school, so I was never saddled with student loans to pay.

As I grew older, I thrived on maintaining autonomy. I lost that during my first marriage when I had to bend to unreasonable demands in order to keep the peace, but I regained it when I left the marriage and made choices that better suited Jessica and me. At that juncture I determined that I'd never again relinquish my autonomy. I reasserted my sense of efficacy and control when Jessica came to live with me after her mom died. I selected her schools and her after-school programs and whom she stayed with when I had to travel for work. And I maintained a strong sense of autonomy after I married Terri because we shared agendas and utter trust in each other. We were a team. She controlled the kitchen and I played the role of sous chef. I kept our finances straight and watered the plants and took out the garbage and helped with groceries and laundry.

Now, how could I keep up my side of the bargain? And what if I'm this way or worse eighteen months from now? From when do I start counting the eighteen months? My spirits drooped like an un-watered tulip as these thoughts flooded my brain. I longed to sleep and dream of miracles and wake up healthy again as I'd been my whole life.

After Dr. Richardson left I thought about the treatments he'd outlined. I had little hope for the plasmapheresis in light of my disappointment with the IVIgG and prednisone treatments that the doctors had been so confident would work. Maybe we should dive headfirst into the Cytoxan. At least there was this study that was somewhat hopeful. Let's not fiddle around with stuff that won't work.

Eighteen months. The clock was ticking.

As I lay back on my bed, I recalled the day several weeks earlier when Drs. Richardson and Kelly had finally reached the tentative diagnosis of CIDP. It had taken two EMG and nerve conduction tests for them to discern damage to the myelin surrounding my nerves. They had been so hopeful that I would make a quick recovery back then. "It's all good news, no bad news," Dr. Kelly had said. Boy was he wrong.

As I pondered these things, I started to doze off. I had slept in fits and starts the previous night, my slumber interrupted by nursing assistants who needed to take my blood pressure or check my temperature. Also, the wailing of distressed patients down the hall didn't help. So I settled back on my pillow, the bed cranked halfway up, but no sooner had I started to doze when one of the interns who had been present during Dr. Richardson's exam knocked on the open door. "I'm sorry to disturb you," she said. "May I give you a neuro exam of my own? I'm studying to be a neurologist. I'd be grateful if you would allow me, although it's strictly up to you."

I was too sleepy to resist. "Okay," I said, and then guided her through it. I'd been through so many of these exams in the preceding weeks and months that I was intimately familiar with the drill and could show off.

When she had finished practicing on me she thanked me, wished me luck and promised to look in on me in the days ahead. After she left, one of the attendants brought me an unappetizing lunch tray: A plain green salad with bits of carrot for color, a dry, leathery sliver of beef with roast potato, and a multi-colored Jell-O ring. I might pick at the Jell-O later. "Just leave it on the dresser," I said.

I slept some and when I awoke I reached for the urinal I kept on the hospital table next to my bed. Since, unlike most patients, I couldn't just hop out of bed to go to the bathroom or retrieve something I wanted that was out of reach, I made sure that certain essential items were always within my grasp. The nurse's call button (which also served as the TV control), my book, a plastic pitcher half filled with water, a stack of Dixie cups, the phone, and the urinal. But I now realized that the aide who had cleaned and straightened my room earlier had put the urinal in the bathroom. So I used the call button to summon the nurse. I hated having to do this for every little thing. I felt envious of other patients who, in varying degrees of bad health, could nevertheless move about the room or the corridors of the hospital pretty much at will.

In about two or three minutes, one of the nurse's aides answered my call. She was the same one who had responded when breakfast was brought and I needed someone to open the packets of sugar for my coffee. By the time she'd come, my coffee was cold. How miserable to be so dependent, especially on strangers. I couldn't wait for the evening when Terri would come straight from work. I felt like a kid. I'd cry on her shoulders and she'd make it all better.

"I'm sorry to bother you," I felt compelled to say to the aide as she entered my room. "But, I need my urinal, it's in the bathroom."

"That's perfectly all right, dear." She brought me an empty and freshly cleaned urinal.

"My condition is temporary," I added, as she hooked the urinal onto the bed rail.

"Of course it is dear," she said. Then she left, and a little while later Dr. Ayles, the energetic head neurology resident, stopped by. I liked him. As the head resident, although young, he was far more experienced and confident in his knowledge than any of the interns or other residents, yet not so full of himself so as to speak condescendingly to patients. I could speak my mind to him and he listened. Also, he alone had found the miracle laxative that worked to unclog my constipated system, a by-product of my immobility. A lemony drink of some sort, Terri and I dubbed it "Dr. Ayles' bombshell."

"I have to get better soon," I whined. "I don't think I can last this way for six months or more."

He was sympathetic, yet practical. "You have suffered a rather severe disability that has come up in a very short time. I've consulted with the senior neurologists and we've agreed that you're a good candidate for Zoloft, an anti-depressant. We'll start you on it now and monitor your dosage carefully. Then you can tell us how it's going."

"Okay," I said, but I was skeptical. I didn't feel that I needed anti-depressant medication despite everything that had befallen me. My anti-depressants were my wife (who had cancelled her upcoming business travel to stay with me), my daughter, the support of my friends and colleagues, and most of all, an unwavering expectation that I would get better someday.

I didn't really want the Zoloft, but the medical advice I got from others was to be open to it. So, I agreed to try it. For goodness sakes, I was already taking more pills than I could count. My whole life I had only taken an Advil or Tylenol now and then. This has to be temporary. Eighteen months. The clock is ticking.

As Dr. Ayles left, the phone rang. I leaned over and tried to pick up the receiver with one hand. The receiver slid to the floor. A tech aide happening by came to the rescue and retrieved it for me. When the phone rang again, I used all my mind power to will my hands into action, and managed to lift the receiver using both hands. It was Terri. "How are you, sweetheart?"

"Tired," I said, "but doing okay. I can't wait to see you." Just hearing her voice cheered me no end.

"I'll be packing up and driving over soon. The office has been very understanding. I'm covered for both trips, and the Court will hear argument by phone in my Seventh Circuit case. How about if I pick up a pizza for dinner?"

"That sounds great," I said, relieved that I wouldn't have to suffer through another hospital meal. It was mid-afternoon and maybe I'd sleep a wink.

Scrap that thought. Beth, my assigned physical therapist, was at the door with a young trainee named Sarah.

"We want to spend the next hour testing your muscles and basically seeing where you're at," Beth said.

"Okay by me, but I think my muscles went AWOL."

Beth was in her mid-twenties, and had a brisk but polite manner. With tastefully applied makeup and shiny brown hair that she wore pulled back in a French knot or bun, she possessed an air of professional confidence that made her seem older than her years. She spoke in a direct, no nonsense manner that made me feel I was in good hands.

Today was assessment day. "First we want to see how you walk using your walker," Beth said, as she tied a safety belt around my waist. Sarah held my belt as I shuffled along the hospital corridor slapping down my legs one at a time. Beth walked along observing my gait.

"For now," Beth said, "I think it best that you not walk alone or without someone holding the safety belt."

"Actually, I've been walking okay with my walker the past couple of days," I said. "I'm not quite so helpless. "

"Bend your knees. It'll hurt your knees to slap the legs down like that," Beth cautioned.

"I can't bend them much," I said.

"Bend," said Beth with each step I took.

"Bend them," echoed Sarah.

We walked the length of the corridor and turned back toward my room. Beth left me in Sarah's hands while she went to retrieve her clipboard that Sarah had forgotten. Sarah, I guessed, was in her early twenties, having recently completed college. She was slightly shorter than Beth with straight blond hair extending just below her shoulders. She explained that she was attending school in California, studying to be a physical therapist. She was interning at GW for the spring semester, and had one month left. She'd be working with me daily and would report to Beth. Sarah was pleasant and upbeat, and I liked her. She could be a little spaced out at times, like forgetting to bring the clipboard and not always keeping track of time. In the days ahead, as we continued to work together, Beth would have occasion to raise her eyebrows or simply shrug at these lapses. But Sarah worked hard with me, and neither Beth nor I could help but like her.

Also, Sarah, like me (or like the old me), was an avid runner. "This must be so hard for you," she said. "I don't know what I'd do if I couldn't run anymore."

"Yes, it is hard, but I expect to get better. Then I'll run again or, if I can't run I'll ride a bike or something."

"The physical therapy will help you over time," Sarah said. I didn't respond; I was skeptical. Therapy alone wouldn't cure me. Still, I couldn't discount the benefit of maintaining what little strength I had left. I guess I'd be wise to accept whatever they tossed my way as an aid in learning to cope with my new world.

We walked back together, and Sarah mistakenly guided me into the room next to mine. The elderly lady who occupied this room seemed oblivious to our intrusion, so we just turned around and slowly made our way back into my room. Beth returned with her clipboard and laughed in disbelief at our faux pas. She then proceeded to administer her own muscle test, similar to those given by the neurologists.

"We'll be back tomorrow and take you to the Physical

Therapy unit for balancing exercises," Beth said at the end of my hour. "In the meantime," she repeated, "you shouldn't walk unaccompanied or without wearing your safety belt." I withheld the urge to protest. "Your muscles are too weak to walk in your condition. You're compensating by leaning hard on the walker with your arms. Most people in your condition wouldn't venture out without a chair."

Before leaving, Beth wanted me to know that if I worked hard at therapy my muscles would adjust, maximizing strength where most needed, so that I could function better. "We will work primarily on balance and bending knees," she said, "and I'll devise a regimen of leg exercises to strengthen your quads and hamstrings. We'll do some walking, but the focus of your therapy will be balance and leg strengthening." Then she engaged me in a little pep talk.

"Most importantly," she said, "you'll have to commit yourself fully to the overall effort. It'll be up to you. I can't work miracles. When you transfer to rehab, which, I understand, may happen next week or the week after, you'll be expected to put in three hours daily for PT and for OT."

"With my condition, the nerves have to be given time to regenerate," I explained. "Unless and until that happens, I don't see therapy making that much of a difference." I remembered how useless the outpatient therapy seemed during the time when I could still walk, but was losing strength steadily.

"From what I've read about your diagnosis—CIDP—it's unclear how long it will take or whether your nerves will recover," Beth said. "In the meantime, therapy can most definitely help your muscles compensate for weaknesses and improve functioning. But you have to be willing to work."

In the weeks and months ahead I would come around to Beth's view, and dedicate myself to the PT sessions with a passion. After all, I was competitive by nature. But now I was torn. My condition was temporary, I'd tell myself. The nerves would regenerate and only then would the muscles work like they had my whole life.

But for the first time, it was dawning on me that I was in for the long haul, and if I were to get better I'd have to work real hard.

I looked at the wall clock. I had but a half-hour to rest until the occupational therapists would come knocking on my door. Then I'd learn creative ways to cope in my strange new world.

6 The Rain Forest

We concocted the scheme to climb Kilimanjaro over beers with our friend Bridgid during a TGIF outing at the Black Cat—a hip bar and club not far from our downtown office. It was late summer 1998, and our conversation turned to the seven summits (the highest peaks on each of the seven continents), and specifically to Kilimanjaro. Bridgid declared that we should all go to Tanzania to climb Kilimanjaro. The expression on her face showed that she meant it and she pleaded for us to agree.

Terri and I had met each other, in part, because we had Bridgid in common. We'd each worked with her in separate places at different times. We knew her to be energetic, athletic and just a little bit mischievous. Petite and slender with short-cropped light brown hair, hazel eyes, and fair skin, she was a magnet for athletic young men. Bridgid and her boyfriend at the time had recently attempted climbing Mt. Whitney in California, but were forced to turn back because of high altitude sickness. They had scrambled—I imagined them racing—to a height of 13,000 feet, and the resulting headaches had forced them to abort their adventure. In addition to her athleticism, Bridgid possessed a singular ability to hold her own with just about any male companion in the hearty enterprise of downing a six-pack.

When Bridgid got an idea into her head, particularly one involving risk and adventure, her eyes would widen and there was no talking her out of it. Indeed, the chances were better that she'd talk you into joining her. So when she said to us in her most earnest voice "let's all go together, let's climb Kilimanjaro," we were hard pressed to refuse. We hesitated at first, as we lacked any mountain climbing experience whatsoever, but by our third beer, Bridgid had convinced us to give it a go.

I cannot honestly put this all on Bridgid, though. I'd become fascinated with mountain climbing stories in recent years. I had been engrossed by *Into Thin Air*, Jon Krakauer's story about the tragic, ill-fated attempt of a group of climbers, some woefully inexperienced, to conquer Everest in the mid-1990s. Also, Terri and I had both just read *Seven Summits*, about the challenge of two wealthy businessmen to reach the summit of the highest mountain of each of the seven continents over a period of several years. Based on their account, we knew that Kilimanjaro was an advanced trek rather than a technical climb of the sort that would mandate use of specialized mountaineering equipment—crampons, ice picks, ropes, and the rest. So, we figured we were in good enough shape to make this trip.

Also, such an adventure would provide a needed escape from the daily grind of our legal employment, a sedentary routine that centered around writing motions, briefs, and memos, attending out of town depositions, and engaging in discovery disputes with opposing counsel over tedious issues such as what categories of documents to produce. By the next summer, as always, we'd need to recharge our batteries, so we agreed to go.

I was also motivated because my newfound athleticism stood in stark contrast to my lack of interest in sports as a kid. Starting when I was nine, for several summers I was sent to a sleep-away camp in the Adirondacks in upstate New York, Brant Lake Camp. A decent swimmer, I earned several patches up to intermediate and was good at track, but anything involving a team, knowing when and where to move or to expect a pass eluded me. I can still see Sammy Applebaum's pockmarked face in mine in the middle of a volleyball game as he hollered "Rotate, you dumb ass."

Camp went well enough until the final week during color war when everyone, even the counselors, got wildly competitive and winning was all that counted. Because I was fast at the 440, the Gray team chose me to run the second leg of the relay my second summer. The relay coach, Uncle Earl, explained that meant reaching back to receive the baton and then, as I finished the leg, passing it to the next runner. "And don't mess up Scadron," he warned, perhaps anticipating that I was likely to do just that. When it was time to line up, Uncle Earl pulled me by my shirt to the block since, as usual, I'd been daydreaming on the sidelines. At the gun I started running and reached behind me for the baton. I could feel the stick grazing my hand but couldn't quite grasp it. It dropped to the ground. Rather than waste precious time picking it up, I continued to run without it. As a result, my team got disqualified and lost to the Green team. I can still recall Uncle Earl, Sammy Applebaum, and what seemed like tens of thousands of angry campers screaming and waving their arms at me. Thank God it was close to the end of camp.

My indifference to athletic achievement could be traced back to my New York upbringing. At home the women dominated. Lou tended to be immersed in his business in Brooklyn where my mother and Pop also worked. So at home it was Ceal, Mom, and us kids. At dinner it was hard for me to get a word in edgewise. The girls yakked and giggled, putting down classmates, particularly boys who didn't pass muster in sophistication or fashion or were otherwise unsuitable as denizens in their world. Lou, my only father figure, was rarely around. When not tending to his business, he'd schmooze with business cronies at the midtown Warwick Hotel Bar.

During my childhood we spent summers in the town of Elberon on the Jersey shore, where my family owned a large Tudor style house on four acres. Arthur, Patsy and I played *Clue*, substituting the rooms in our house for the rooms on the game board and the members of my family for the potential suspects and victims. It might be Uncle Lou or Pop who did it in the ballroom with the candlestick, instead of Colonel Mustard. It was mostly during these summers that I saw Arthur, my oldest childhood friend. Our families were close, and his folks had a house in the neighboring town of Deal. We played ball, biked around town, swam in the ocean, and frolicked on the boardwalk in Asbury Park.

Unlike me, Arthur was athletic, excelling at most sports. He was also a smart aleck. We'd play catch on the sprawling front lawn. "Go way back," he'd holler, as he threw the baseball way over my head knowing full well how poor my judgment was when it came to flagging down a fly ball. He had me running ragged. Occasionally on weekends, Lou and my mother would take the train down from the city. Sometimes, while relaxing on the front porch, they'd observe us at play. "He throws like a girl," Lou continually said of me. But he never took the time to teach me any other way.

Perhaps the event that more than anything else transformed me from city slicker to outdoor adventurer occurred in the mid-1970's when I went hiking in the Idaho wilderness area with my buddy Bob from law school and his wife Doris. I'd gotten to know them both quite well, and I rented a room in the house where they lived during our second and third year at George Washington University. Doris, about a year older than us, was working as a paralegal for a small law office.

With his uncombed hair flopping every which way, Bob intensely involved himself in any activity he undertook: hiking, running, backyard basketball, downing a six-pack, even hitting the law books. Whenever he told a story, his eyes bulged and he became animated. But he was a good listener and always opinionated. If he didn't like what I had to say, he'd damn well let me know, or he'd just as vigorously agree with me.

Doris, petite with dark hair, light skin and freckles, had a bubbly, infectious personality. She seemed to bring out the best in Bob.

After law school, Bob and Doris married and then drove across country, settling in Boise where the mountains and open spaces offered plenty of opportunity for the outdoor life they both loved. Bob joined a law firm and Doris worked on and off at odd jobs.

I planned a three-week western road trip that summer of '76, working in visits with friends in San Francisco and Seattle. Boise seemed as good a place to start as any. So I phoned Bob proposing a weekend visit. He became excited about the prospect of camping with Doris and me in the mountains, something I'd hardly ever done.

Until I broke away from my childhood home after college and established my own identity, I was the epitome of a city slicker. My primary act of rebellion was to walk everywhere if feasible. Most of all it was Bob who influenced me during our years in law school to take up running and hiking in the woods. His world was as different from the one I'd grown out of as a poodle is from a squirrel.

So I became excited when Bob revealed his plan for my upcoming visit. He and Doris had spent time hiking in the Sawtooths, a group of mountains known for their sharp, rugged peaks. But Bob wanted to show me the more remote wilderness area of north central Idaho. If we got lucky, we might see eagles, falcon, elk, and the elusive mountain goats.

I brought with me a full size backpack, a sleeping bag, hiking boots, a poncho, a canteen that could hold a liter of water, and a pillow. "You brought a pillow!" Bob bellowed. "You might as well have brought a teddy bear."

"I did bring my favorite stuffed animal," I said, and Bob let out a loud guffaw before I could add, "just kidding."

We started out at dusk and drove north for four hours, the last hour over dirt roads before we reached the head of the trail. We positioned our sleeping bags to avoid sharp stones and hoped for four hours of sleep before dawn. I didn't get any even with my pillow.

We began our hike at daybreak, climbing thousands of feet through forest and meadows, occasionally crossing narrow brooks. The air was cool but the sun beat down on me with a vengeance, and I continually had to remove my glasses to wipe sweat from my brow. At a good stopping point, Doris pulled out a red and black scarf from her pack and fixed a bandana for me to wear. My pack felt heavy—damn pillow—so I removed the pack even though we'd only be able to rest for five minutes or so. "That's a mistake," Doris said, and I soon realized how right she was when the time came to move on, and I had to heave the pack back over my aching shoulders.

Bob carried a detailed topography map of the area that he referred to frequently. He'd selected a campsite by a high alpine lake. The plan was to stop for lunch at one of the many lakes that dotted the region, after which we'd descend several thousand feet before climbing again. When we started to descend, some of the terrain was quite steep. Bob showed me how to maneuver downhill safely over uneven ground. "Go down sideways like this," he said, "always keep your first foot in front, never cross your feet and always, always lean uphill. Watch me." I did as I was shown.

We'd trekked for nine hours altogether, uphill and down, before reaching our site at four in the afternoon. We didn't come across a soul all day, unless small mammals and birds have souls. With relief I removed my pack and collapsed on my sleeping bag. When I looked up, Bob and Doris had already pitched the tent. "That's something you must absolutely do right away or you won't do it at all," she explained. "We've learned that from experience."

"Who wants to swim?" Bob asked. "I do," I said, "but I didn't bring a suit."

"Oh, for gosh sakes, swim in your underpants," Doris laughed. "No one will mind here."

Bob and I dashed into the lake, and never did such frigid water feel so good. Still, I only lasted five minutes. Bob stayed in for almost half an hour, while Doris busied herself arranging stuff inside the tent. I slept well that night.

The next day grew cloudy as we took several walks in different directions, always keeping an eye out for goats. We saw a Peregrine falcon, a rare sighting Bob said, and heard what sounded to him like a bugling elk, but no goats.

That night it stormed like a demon. The sky opened up with a deluge and water leaked into an open seam on my side of the tent. I repositioned my bag as best I could, which was not good enough. After a long while Bob woke up and zipped up the seam. In the meantime, my pillow and some belongings got soaked. "You should have woken us," Doris said in the morning.

After a breakfast of bread and cereal, we packed up, donned our ponchos, and set out for the long journey back down the mountain. I had no choice but to leave my heavy, soggy pillow behind, all too aware that I was littering this pristine environment. I hoped the elusive goats might come across it some day and be grateful for a ready place to bed down.

We made it back to Boise intact and promised each other we'd find goats another time. My transformation from city slicker to outdoorsman was now complete and set the stage for other adventures, although my Kilimanjaro climb wouldn't happen for another couple of decades.

After making our pact with Bridgid at the Black Cat, Terri and I engaged the services of a company specializing in Africa, primarily safaris and Kilimanjaro climbs. We planned to spend the first week on safari, working in a supervised hike at 8000 feet (in an area safe from lions, leopard, cape buffalo and other wildlife you wouldn't care to meet), in order to help us acclimate to the altitude. Kilimanjaro rises 19,000 feet into the African sky. We would need to adequately prepare if we were to avoid the main risk: high altitude sickness. We'd devote the second week to the climb and spend the final week of the trip recuperating on the sprawling white beaches of Zanzibar Island.

Despite her apparent initial enthusiasm, Bridgid did not make the trip with us. "I have to act really, really fast on a tempting job opportunity back home in Minnesota," she explained. So she apologetically bowed out of the trip. Just as well, we figured, as she would have set a torrid pace—too fast for us and for her own good. Instead, our tour company hooked us up with a couple from Chicago, Lisa and Ray, who, as it turned out, were a good match for us.

We met Lisa and Ray the evening before the climb at the Mountain Village Inn, a small resort just outside of Arusha, Tanzania's second largest city and gateway to Kilimanjaro. Like us, they had booked rooms at this resort for the day before and the day after the climb. In Chicago, they both worked in finance at a large banking institution. In their mid-forties, they appeared trim and fit, but, thank goodness, not super athletic. On their flight over, Lisa's luggage had been lost, and the tour company did its best to find replacement items that she'd need for the climb. "There is one item that they have not replaced which we cannot do without, and we are hoping you guys can help."

"What is that?" Terri asked.

"Toilet paper," Lisa whispered.

"Oh, we have oodles of toilet paper," Terri said reassuringly. "We can divvy it up tomorrow."

Mountain Village consisted of a cluster of bungalows set amid a coffee plantation. The dwellings, overlooking a scenic lake, were surrounded by gardens of passion fruit, mango, and banana trees. After we arrived, Terri and I hiked part way around the lake with an employee of the hotel named James. James promised to treat us to a banana beer when we got back if we had successfully reached the summit. I wasn't sure what a banana beer was exactly, but my hunch was that it was considerably more potent than Budweiser.

The next morning our safari guide, Rasoul, drove Ray, Lisa, Terri and me to within one mile of our starting point at the Machame gate. There are many routes up Kilimanjaro. We chose Machame because it was not as popular (and crowded) as the Marengo route, a little tougher but not beyond our ability. We heard that the Marengo route was most popular with the beer and pretzel crowd, while Machame was meant for the wine and cheese set. So Machame seemed to fit us best anyway. When Rasoul dropped us off one mile short of the Machame gate, he explained that the road beyond would be too mucky and steep for the Land Rover. The bonus mile would serve as a warm up for the ambitious journey we were about to undertake.

The land around us was partially forested with wide stretches of cultivated fields on both sides. Trudging toward the park entrance, we could see coffee and a variety of fruits grown on these lower slopes of the mountain. Small houses dotted the cultivated fields, while vendors selling soft drinks, beer, and snacks of pine nuts, peanuts, and jerky, lined the dirt road. Gradually, the forest grew thicker, with vines and moss forming a thick canopy overhead, blocking out the sun.

We each carried daypacks and a ski pole that we'd been issued to use as a walking stick. I wore shorts, my Sabi Sabi T-shirt (from the game reserve in South Africa where I had stayed a few years earlier), and my new hiking boots I'd purchased back in Washington at REI, a store that catered to outdoor enthusiasts. In the days ahead I would add layers of clothing now tucked away in my duffel. We were starting out at 6,000 feet, and the first day would take us uphill through rain forest to 10,000 feet. The plains below the mountain are about 3,000 feet in elevation, so the morning drive saved us 3,000 feet of climbing. We would take five days to reach the summit according to our itinerary. Most groups take four days but we requested an extra day to help assure that we'd acclimate to the high altitude. An additional two days was relegated to the descent that would follow a steeper trail than the one going up.

Even before reaching the park entrance, the going was muddy and slippery, and before long my shoes were caked in mud. "Great start, considering that we won't be showering for a whole seven days," I moaned.

"Just wait until the end of today," Lisa said. "I have a feeling that the going will be wetter and more slippery as we go through the forest."

At the gate we hooked up with our guide, James, and our team of 11 porters, all just for the four of us. Freelance trekking is prohibited on Kilimanjaro. Regulations require that each climbing group be assigned a team of porters. Throughout the trek, the porters would carry our duffels, tents, food, and drink, always on their heads. This included baskets of eggs. (I guess they figured that Americans could not do without their eggs for breakfast, not even for one week). The porters generally wore T-shirts, shorts and sandals. No walking sticks for them. One of our porters sported a N.Y. Yankees cap, a man after my own heart.

As climbers, we were hardly alone. Other groups from all over the world were also assembled at the gate registering for the climb. We posed for photos in front of the large brown sign marking the park entrance. The sign presented a list of "Points to Remember:"

"Hikers attempting to reach the summit should be physically fit. If you have a sore throat, cold or breathing problems don't go above 3,000 meters. Drink 4-5 liters of fluid every day."

"That's an awful lot of water," Ray said.

"If signs of mountain sickness or high altitude diseases persist please descend immediately."

Those were just a couple of the caveats.

"Should we descend now?" Terri asked.

As soon as we passed through the gate we were trekking steadily uphill through lush and misty jungle. There were palms and lichen and mosses hanging from tree limbs. Tree ferns grew to at least 20 feet high. This was an utterly new landscape for me, yet it was hard to fully appreciate the eerie beauty of the scene as the slippery and, at times, steep course took all my concentration.

As we set out, I'd made a mental note to keep my eyes peeled for the white and black Colobus monkeys that our book said could be seen in the forest. But instead of looking around, I found myself ascending muddy slopes by grabbing onto tree limbs and pulling myself along, keeping my eyes glued to the ground below. Of the four of us, I encountered the greatest difficulty. I slipped, tumbled, got all muddy, and cursed.

"What's the trouble, Michael?" James asked, concerned after I took perhaps my third or fourth spill of the day. James was a short but sturdy and powerfully built Tanzanian native with a stern demeanor. I wanted to stay on his good side.

"It's just slippery," I said.

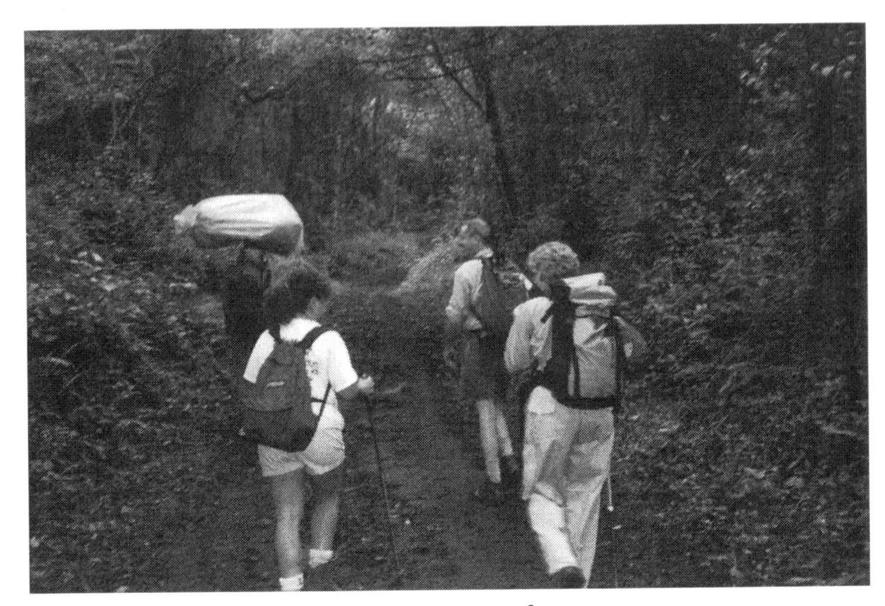

Hiking in the rain forest

We continued to slog and pull our way through the rain forest, occasionally falling behind, but sometimes moving ahead of other climbers. “Slow and steady,” I told myself. *“Polé polé,”* the porters chanted—their Swahili term for “Slowly, slowly”. Muddied trousers and shoes provided comforting assurance that I was not the only one on the mountain that day awkwardly groping and sliding my way uphill. One heavyset woman we met along the way was so covered in mud from head to toe she resembled a bathing baby hippo at a watering hole. I later learned that she gave up on the ordeal after the second day.

The mist grew thicker by late afternoon, making for a spooky, yet enchanting scene. I imagined a war movie set in a jungle of some distant land. We were soldiers on the move, weary from the long march, but vigilant lest the enemy appear, suddenly, from out of the fog. No monkeys graced us with their presence that day. Probably just as well, as they would have howled with laughter at my clumsiness.

We didn’t reach camp until nightfall. Exhausted and dirty, I lost my bearing and fell in the mud several more times before emerging from the rain forest. James looked back now and then with a worried expression, but he said little more. James was a man of few words. I'm sure by day's end he'd assigned us, particularly me, little chance of reaching the summit. When we finally arrived at camp, the porters set up our tent and brought food and drink, while we, brave souls, collapsed on our sleeping bags. I looked forward to the morning when, having said good bye and good riddance to the rain forest, we would enter the drier lower alpine zone, a region characterized by giant heather, scattered bushes, and delicate flowers of all colors.

Most folks that I have spoken to who have successfully climbed Kilimanjaro recall the final ascent to the top at night as the most difficult part of the climb. Being awakened at 11 p.m., after just a few winks of sleep, to brave wind and freezing temperatures to reach the summit by early morning, and then to immediately descend to first camp at 10,000 feet, is certainly a daunting challenge. I may be alone, however, in recalling the first day of the climb through the muddy rain forest as the toughest part of the entire Kilimanjaro experience.

Years later, as I recalled the rain forest to a friend, he remarked that perhaps I'd already been experiencing the first symptoms of my neuropathy. My first clear symptoms didn't occur until about four months after we got home, so the time sequence is highly unlikely. Moreover, if his hypothesis were true, it was something of a miracle that I didn't have to be carried off the mountain on a stretcher.

7 Jessica's Mountain

If Terri and I had been in a state of denial in the days following my diagnosis in February of 2000, Jessica was not. She was frightened, only I was too blind to notice. Even when her high school guidance counselor phoned me at home, I couldn't see what should have been obvious, especially in light of her childhood traumas.

"Hello, Mr. Scadron, this is Ms. Landsman. How are you doing?"

"I'm okay," I said. "How are you?"

"I'm fine really. The reason I'm calling is that Jessica has expressed her concern—in fact, she is really very worried about your health. She talks about you every day and, frankly, she is quite distraught. We are hesitant to reassure her because we don't know what your medical situation is. I don't mean to pry, but because of Jessica's stress, that's why I'm calling."

"I'll talk to her," I said. I explained the doctors had assured me that the treatments they prescribed should help me get better soon, maybe even within a few weeks. "Jessica shouldn't worry," I insisted. "I'll talk to her tonight. Thanks for letting me know."

"Okay, Mr. Scadron, we'd be grateful if you would. Certainly, we all wish you the best."

Jessica was in her senior year at Chelsea in Silver Spring, a special needs school for youngsters with learning disabilities. She was to graduate in June, and I was proud of her for having come this far. She had endured a series of upheavals in her young life that had contributed to low self-esteem and made her vulnerable: difficulties with schoolwork, a volatile relationship between her parents, followed by a nasty divorce. And she had to watch helplessly as her mother wasted away from incurable brain cancer when Jessica was eight. No wonder she was now so worried about me, notwithstanding my assurances that I would get better.

Jessica recalls taking a walk with her mom in Rock Creek Park, just a few blocks from their Mount Pleasant house near the zoo. It was during the summer of 1989, several months after Sylvia had undergone surgery to remove a malignant brain tumor. Jessica was then eight, and her mom and I had been living apart for about three years.

Sylvia used to go for early morning jogs in the park, but, after the surgery, she satisfied herself with brisk walks. At some point mother and daughter sat down on a bench to rest. It looked to Jessica like her mom was blowing bubbles. She soon realized that her mom was having a seizure and that it was foam, not bubbles, oozing from her mouth. Jessica had seen these seizures before. She knew she'd have to get help. She tried waving down bikers and runners, but failed to catch their attention. Finally, a Latino woman took notice and gave Sylvia and Jessica a ride back to their house. Once back at home, Jessica went to get the help of Robyn, a friend who lived a block away.

Robyn made soup for Sylvia and held her hand. Sylvia insisted on keeping with her plan to take Jessica swimming. Hour-long swims had helped calm Sylvia's moods somewhat, and on our travels abroad, we had always searched for a pool so that she might spend the mornings swimming while I watched or swam with Jessica. Even having suffered this seizure, Sylvia remained insistent on going for her swim. Robyn persuaded her to imagine instead that the bowl of soup was a swimming pool.

When Sylvia and I married in 1978, we moved into a small Victorian-era row house in the Mount Pleasant neighborhood of

D.C. Mount Pleasant is an enclave of row houses mostly dating to the 1920's and earlier, with mature trees shading its narrow residential streets. It is nestled between hectic Mount Pleasant Street with its taverns, shops, and eateries to the east, and then slopes down to the Rock Creek Park bike path that parallels the backside of the National Zoo to the west. When we lived there, the neighborhood was becoming transitional with yuppies buying and renovating properties previously occupied by blacks and Hispanics. A friend who lived in the relatively peaceful side near the park referred to the area adjoining Mount Pleasant Street as the "war zone." We lived in the war zone.

In time, Sylvia quit her government job, for which she had little aptitude and no patience, and took up painting, for which she had a great deal of talent. Her paintings, many of which were psychological portraits of family members and acquaintances, offered a glimpse of the demons that haunted her soul.

Trespassers depicts several friends of ours, each recognizable, just outside the front door to our house, peering in through the windows. Their heads are exaggerated in size and their facial expressions distorted into sinister smiles or glares. Sylvia herself is standing inside the house sketching or taking notes.

Cowlady, completed in the year Jessica was born, is a self-portrait in which the artist stands naked and obviously pregnant, her features contorted, on an English hillside on the southern coast of Cornwall, overlooking the English Channel. The colors are rich and vibrant—golden green grass against a deep blue sea. A large black and white cow stands directly behind her grazing on the grass. One of her artist friends remarked that, when viewing this painting, she didn't know whether to laugh or cry.

There were some signs early on in our relationship that Sylvia had a volatile temperament, but I didn't gauge the full extent of her condition. When we married she had been estranged from her family for many years and our efforts to reunite with them proved difficult. Gradually, I learned that her mother, who came from England, was a mean-spirited woman who had taken pleasure in pitting Sylvia and her younger sisters against one another. Her father suffered from bouts of alcoholism. On occasion Sylvia would startle me by storming out of the house in a fit of rage, seemingly over nothing. Later, when she'd calmed down, she'd explain that she had suffered a transference, that unconsciously she had redirected her childhood anger onto me. I was attracted to her because she had good insights gained by years of experience in psychotherapy. She was extraordinarily creative, though short on logic and the ability to engage in calm deliberation.

We shared good times early in our marriage: going to the theater and art museums, driving into the neighboring countryside, entertaining friends in our home, cooking together, and taking summer holidays abroad. But the ups and downs of Sylvia's moods soon began to weigh on me and made it difficult for me to fully love her the way I'd hoped I would.

Looking back now, I know there were telltale signs that should have warned me that I'd be out of my depth in marrying Sylvia, that she was too complicated for me, too fragile. A more mature man might be able to provide the nurturing and patience that such a relationship required. But my inexperience with women contributed to an immaturity that prevented me from foreseeing the demands that such a marriage would involve or from recognizing my inability to make the necessary commitment.

I took pride in Sylvia's painting, but I had plenty of sleepless nights worrying about how we could survive on my salary alone. I also grew weary of her tantrums, which became more frequent after Jessica was born. During the time when we were attempting to preserve our marriage through counseling, a psychiatrist—a family practitioner—suggested that Sylvia likely had a bipolar mood disorder and would benefit from medication. He offered to monitor her on a trial of lithium. She refused, fearing that medication would curb her creativity. "This is what these shrinks prescribe in order to shut women up," she said.

I sorely wanted a calmer environment for Jessica and me. But when I suggested that medication might help her better focus on her work and lead to greater productivity, she became enraged. More and more, if I didn't provide unconditional support for whatever it was that she thought she needed, she got angry and said that I wasn't a supportive or nurturing husband. And increasingly, as her demands became greater and less reasonable, I found it impossible to provide the unconditional support that she wanted. So we fought. We shouted. Objects flew across the room like missiles. She'd slap me and in frustration I'd punch one of her paintings, while Jessica watched.

By the time Jessica turned three, she still hadn't spoken a word. We took her for a full battery of tests. The resulting diagnosis was "developmental delays"—across the board. She also demonstrated poor behavior and impulse control. We sought and received funding to have her placed in special needs schooling. She switched schools several times before we got her into Ivymount in Rockville, Maryland, an excellent placement for kids with learning disabilities and a variety of other issues, albeit not for emotional disturbances.

In the meantime, Sylvia became more reclusive and her tantrums increased in intensity and frequency. When I left in the morning to catch the bus to work, I felt like a prisoner being let out of his cell for the day on a work-release program. Then in the evening I'd come home not knowing what to expect. Typically, Sylvia would retreat to the attic to paint, instructing me to put Jessica to bed and then fix dinner.

One evening I came home, read Jessica a bedtime story after feeding and bathing her, and then came downstairs to the kitchen to make a dinner of chicken and rice. Around eight o'clock, I called Sylvia to come down to eat, but she ignored me. After a while, I went upstairs to her attic studio to nudge her to come down. She hollered at me to get out. I went back down to the kitchen and finally around ten o'clock she came down. She screamed at me that the dinner was over-cooked and threw the pot of rice straight at me. Jessica peered from the top of the stairs to get a birds-eye view of the commotion. I don't think we ate anything for dinner that night. I slept downstairs in the basement.

My presence in the same home was not helping the cause of family stability. We occasionally took trips abroad, to England and France, but those only served as temporary escapes. In her attic studio, where she spent so much of her time, Sylvia painted portraits of people from photos taken during those trips, powerful paintings in which she exaggerated the idiosyncrasies of the British or French people who were, unwittingly, the object of her art. She showed her paintings through a cooperative art gallery in downtown Washington. *The Washington Post* gave her work a rave review—calling one of her works "masterful"—but she didn't sell enough paintings to cover the art supplies. The financial pressures grew.

She balked if I wanted to see friends or do anything on my own. "You can take care of Jessica while I'm swimming," an impractical demand in light of my work schedule. Or, "Why don't you leave government and get a real job with a law firm so you can support my art work and we can afford a nanny, like Mark and Betsy."

One Easter, Arthur and Liz came down from their home in New Jersey to visit. Sylvia didn't want them staying with us—"I don't want them butting in"—so they took a hotel room. Arthur and Liz knew that I was unhappy in my marriage. I hadn't said anything to them outright, but they could sense it. After they got to town, they came to the house to say hello. I answered the door, and we greeted each other warmly. Sylvia was upstairs in her studio. At once, she started screaming. "How rude. Who do these people think they are, barging in like this. Tell them to leave at once."

For a while we ignored Sylvia's rants, continuing to chat and visit by the front door, but not for long. Within moments, she came storming downstairs in a rage, gesturing wildly and demanding that the intruders get out. Arthur and Liz hurriedly bid me good-bye and left. Perhaps it was paranoia, or some other obsession, but just as Sylvia had depicted our acquaintances in her artwork, she saw Arthur and Liz as trespassers, larger than life.

I felt as trapped as a white water rafter choosing between steep, dangerous falls directly ahead or facing a family of grizzlies on the shore. How could I leave the marital home and abandon my daughter to the care of a woman whose emotional needs were so great that she'd be unable to meet Jessica's? And then there was the money issue. How could I afford rent for myself on top of our mortgage when there was already barely enough money to pay the bills? On the other hand, how could I stay in that house? My presence had become a trigger for more frequent and prolonged outbursts. My staying there was not helping Jessica one bit. Leaving was my only option.

Jessica was four when I finally left the house, rented a basement apartment down the street, and filed for divorce.

On the day I left, I went to Jessica's school to speak with the director and explain the situation at home. She wasn't surprised. She had seen enough to sense that Sylvia suffered from volatile mood swings. She implored me to stay in Jessica's life no matter what the hardship. I assured her in no uncertain terms that I would.

Sylvia made repeated demands for money that I could not meet. Accusations flew like bullets at a firing range. She didn't want me to see Jessica because I might hurt the child in some way. Through my lawyer, I asked for and got a court-appointed mental health professional to evaluate the situation and mediate a visitation schedule. Even then, however, Sylvia adhered to her own schedule, one that suited her moods. Many times she called or left notes for me at the last minute. "Jessica can't see you tonight because we have to go to an art opening," or "Take Jessica this morning instead of next weekend because I want to go for a swim." The visits became unpredictable, and Jessica, like any child, yearned for predictability.

On one occasion when I went to pick up Jessica for a regular Tuesday evening visit, her mother refused to let me in the house. Jessica came outside, pulled at her mother's dress, stomped her feet, hollered, and cried, all to no avail. I felt helpless. I desperately wanted to end the hostility for Jessica's sake. While remaining in the house hadn't been a viable option, I was determined to stay connected to my daughter. So I worked with my therapists and the social workers and teachers at Ivymount to at least try to do what was best for Jessica. I don't think anyone knew all the right answers.

Finally, Sylvia and I were divorced, but her erratic and volatile behavior persisted when I tried to visit with Jessica, and it was clear to me that the situation was affecting Jessica's behavior at school. She was acting out, the teachers said. She was going on seven by now, in her second year at Ivymount. The school director asked that we arrange for independent counseling for her and said that we'd have to look for a more appropriate placement for the following year, a school that could better address Jessica's emotional concerns. We never reached that point. Sylvia's illness interceded.

It was on a Sunday, just before Christmas of 1988, when I first noticed something physically amiss with Sylvia. I'd taken Jessica to St. Margaret's Church on Connecticut Avenue to help make ornaments for the upcoming Christmas pageant. We were waiting outside at the appointed hour for Sylvia to fetch Jessica. As she arrived, I could see that her upper body was slightly stooped over to one side like she was trying to shake water out of her ear. A couple of days later she told me that she had Lyme disease and would be checking into Georgetown Hospital.

The following week, I took Jessica to the hospital to visit her mom. While I was waiting outside the room I noticed the medical fact sheet pertaining to Sylvia posted on a board just outside her room. The term brain tumor leaped out at me. I must have looked confused because a nurse rushed over to me. "Can I help you, sir?"

"Yes, I think so. I'm this woman's husband. We're divorced but our daughter is here visiting. My understanding is that she had a diagnosis of Lyme..."

"I'll get the doctor. Please wait here."

The doctor explained that they had suspected Lyme disease but that an MRI showed the tumor. The surgery that morning had been partially successful, but the tumor was malignant. It had fingers that extended out from the core and they hadn't been able to remove all of it. He said that it was a slow growing tumor and that the patient might survive anywhere from six months to a year.

I was floating in space, a hundred disconnected thoughts swirling through my mind. My world, and Jessica's, was about to change dramatically, yet again. Death had never become so personal for me before.

I'd enjoyed my time as a carefree single person before I married

Sylvia, meeting friends for dinner or the theater, arranging pick-up basketball games with work buddies at the "Y" or an outdoor court, dating occasionally. I lost these associations after we married, as Sylvia's demands on my time increased and her uneven temperament made it hard to spend time with friends. After Jessica was born, instead of growing into my role as a father, I became a prisoner to my wife's whims, my autonomy altogether lost. After our separation and divorce, I slowly began to regain a sense of control and purpose, as I strived to be a positive force in my daughter's life. Now, this sudden turn of events would take me in an entirely different direction than the one I had expected. Suddenly, I was about to become a single father, someone who needed to create a calm and safe environment for my daughter while balancing the demands of work and family life. Could I do it?

When Jessica's visit with her mom ended, I took her hand and somehow we made it through the halls, down the elevator, across the hospital grounds and back to the car. She didn't know it yet, but I was all she'd have to guide her through her remaining school years. It would fall entirely on me to keep her safe, and to help her overcome the obstacles that she'd faced and the trauma still to come. *In all of this, I must not fail.*

In the weeks ahead I tried to learn more about Sylvia's condition, but it became clear that she didn't want most people, and particularly me, to know that her prognosis was terminal. Instead, she maintained that her condition was hopeful. Even her close friends were left to wonder.

Her mother, known to Jessica as Grandma Edna, flew out to stay with her, and in June they traveled to Amsterdam for an exhibit of Sylvia's artwork while Jessica stayed with me. Sylvia's recent paintings revealed a darker side. The Dracula series, which included three new works, portrayed contorted visions of herself, Jessica, and me as vampires or vampire victims. The backdrop was Whitby Abbey in the town of Whitby on a hill overlooking the northeast seacoast of England. In the novel by Bram Stoker, Whitby was where Dracula had settled when he came to England from Transylvania. Sylvia and I had traveled there with Jessica on one of our trips a few years back. I recognized the ruins of the abbey from our photos.

Sylvia and her mother returned from Amsterdam in late June, earlier than expected. Apparently, Sylvia's seizures had become more frequent. I returned Jessica to the care of her mom, but within a day or two she was back with me. Sylvia, once again, had been admitted to Georgetown Hospital. She remained in the hospital for several weeks. The doctors attempted a procedure known as a shunt, but without success. Sylvia didn't regain consciousness. Jessica's assigned social worker at Ivymount, Sheri, pressed me for information, but I had been kept outside the medical consultations and had little insight to offer.

Some weeks later Sylvia was transferred to a hospice in the Cleveland Park neighborhood, not far from where I lived. She was fed through tubes. I took my daughter there to see her several times a week. By then it was clear to everyone that she was dying. I talked with therapists and teachers on the matter of how and when to break the news to Jessica. Sheri graciously came to our apartment several times over the next several weeks to help me in that difficult undertaking. During the first session, we sat down on the sofa and told Jessica that her mother was dying.

"It might be weeks or it might be months," Sheri said. "But there is very little chance that your mom will regain consciousness. I'm so sorry, Jessica, but your mom is going to die." Sheri was emphatic. The consensus by all the people I trusted to know such things was that Jessica should be given the news in no uncertain terms.

Jessica cried for several minutes. Then she wanted to know what would happen to her. "You will continue to live with me," I said. "We will find a bigger place so that we each have our own room. And you will continue to go to Ivymount." These assurances calmed her.

Grandma Edna was furious about our having told Jessica that Sylvia was dying. She'd told Jessica repeatedly that her mom would get better. "Jessica told her mother that you told her she was going to die. And her mother understood because I could see her move her head. Don't you dare tell her that again."

"I'm working with the therapists and teachers to help Jessica start the grieving process. We're acting in Jessica's best interest," I said.

Following two months of hospice care, Sylvia died on October 5, 1989. "At last she's at peace," her younger sister said to me over the phone.

I felt sad, but that sadness was coupled with relief, overwhelming relief. And hope. Hope that Jessica could begin to flourish in a calm and stable home. Whatever love I may have felt toward Sylvia had dissipated in the course of our tumultuous marriage and breakup. Her constant tantrums and mood swings, exhibited long before her illness, had taken a toll on Jessica as well as me. Jessica and her mom had been close, maybe too close. I'd feared greatly for Jessica's future. As she grew up, would she be permitted an independent sense of identity? Would she be allowed to hang with her own set of friends? Or would that make her mom jealous? I had worried that Jessica's own needs might be subrogated to her mom's enormous and all-consuming emotional needs.

Jessica had turned eight in August, while her mother was in hospice care. We'd celebrated her birthday by throwing her a party at an ice cream parlor in Rockville, not far from her school, a place where sirens rang each time the servers brought out a birthday cake. An odd mix of folks had come: Edna, some of Jessica's classmates, a few of Sylvia's friends, and some of my friends. Foreign worlds colliding.

When I got the call from Edna that Sylvia had died, I left work, took the metro home, got the car, and drove up to Ivymount. The teachers pulled Jessica out of class and sat with me as I broke the news to her. After she had a good long cry, we went outdoors where her classmates were having recess. I took my daughter's hand as her homeroom teacher led us past the playground area and past a cluster of pine trees to a more private grassy expanse behind the school. It was a crisp fall day and the leaves on some of the trees were starting to change color. A teacher's aide rounded up Jessica's seven classmates and they followed us. Her classmates gathered around her in a semi-circle as she explained the news to them. After she told them her mommy had died, one girl came over and gave her a hug. Several others said "I'm sorry, Jessica." Then I took her by the hand and we drove home.

Jessica participated in the memorial service for Sylvia at St. Margaret's Church, carrying the box containing Sylvia's ashes to a stone vault carved into a wall of the sanctum. Doing this helped afford an outlet for her grief. The Reverend Vienna Anderson had explained to Jessica that the ashes came from a very hot fire; that her mom would never come back to earth, but would be with her in spirit always.

Jessica came to live with me in my small one-bedroom condo on Connecticut Avenue. I made a special effort to be there for her. I'd leave work a half hour early to fetch her from her after school program, I'd fix dinners nightly, and, together, we planned activities on weekends. I knew this would be a fragile time for her. Not surprisingly, and not because of anything special that I did, she gradually stopped acting out in school, and, for the first time, started to read. Her handwriting improved markedly. She paid attention in class, minded her teachers and participated in special events. "Thank you for giving us back Jessica," her music teacher told me about two months into the new school year.

After I sold the Mount Pleasant house, I sold the one-bedroom condo on Connecticut Avenue and bought a two-bedroom unit in the same building. Most of the artwork that Jessica inherited was rolled up for storage. A few paintings were still in frames and we hung those in our new apartment. I stashed a few loose pieces under my bed, and there were a few sleepless nights when the bed would creak and moan. Finding a venue for the artwork would someday be a father-daughter project.

In my years as a single dad I dated, but had little interest in remarrying. My first marriage had left me exhausted and I needed time to recover. Also, I wanted to concentrate on being Mr. Mom to Jessica.

Being the parent of a special needs kid entailed, among other things, attending twice-yearly meetings at the school to discuss my daughter's progress and other issues that may have arisen with her team of teachers and to sign off on an Individual

Education Plan (IED) for the following year. I recall one such meeting in particular.

I enter the school and find Jessica's fourth grade classroom. The table and chairs are low to the ground, suitable for nine-year olds but challenging for adults. Seated around the table, waiting for me, are Jessica's three homeroom teachers, her occupational therapist, language therapist, assigned social worker, and Mrs. Davis, the assistant principal.

"Welcome, Mr. Scadron. Before we get started, there is one item we need to address," said Mrs. Bir, the main homeroom teacher. "Jessica told her friend Mark that she'd peeked into your bedroom when your friend Barbara was staying over one weekend and saw the two of you, you know...."

Uh oh, at this point I'm starting to perspire and it's not on account of the temperature.

"Apparently," Mrs. Bir continued, "this upset Mark very much and he cried and hollered at home and so his mother asked that we raise the matter with you. There's no need to discuss this further, just next time be more careful, maybe lock your door."

I tried to mentally reconstruct what happened. I had been seeing Barbara since a short while before Sylvia had died. Jessica was ten, and we were then living in our new two-bedroom condo on upper Connecticut Avenue. Barbara occasionally stayed over on weekends. The past couple of weekends, after Jessica's bedtime, we'd fooled around and had sex in bed. My bedroom door closed, but not real tight and it had no lock. Jessica must have woken up, opened the door a crack, and peeked in without our knowing.

As I drove home after the meeting, which, thank God, was otherwise uneventful, I wondered whether to say anything to Jessica. I decided not to, at least not right away. As it turned out, I didn't need to. "Dad," she greeted me, "I know how you grown ups did it in the sixties." She must have realized the matter would be brought up with me at the school meeting. We had a little chat.

Jessica remained at Ivymount for several more years. She thrived enough there that she was able to switch schools in the fall of 1993 to one with a less restrictive setting.

Barbara and I eventually broke off our relationship. She wanted to get married but I wasn't ready. In fact, it took several more years before I was ready, once again, to venture into a lasting relationship. Then, when I turned fifty, I met Terri. Timing is everything. One year earlier, Terri and I might not have meshed.

When I met Terri, Jessica had turned 15, the age of resistance. "You guys are loony," she told me when I asked her if she could accept Terri as a stepmom. It was obvious that she felt suddenly threatened by what had developed into a serious relationship for me.

"You know Dad, I've been thinking," she said to me after school one day. "Remember how you used to tell me that you might remarry, and if you did, the woman you chose might act like my mother but wouldn't ever take the place of my real mother?"

"Sure, I remember those talks after your mom died."

"Well, I've given it a lot of thought since you've been going out with Terri. To be perfectly honest, I've kinda gotten used to it just being you and me."

"Jessica, you'll always be with me even if Terri and I get married," I said, but I could tell she wasn't so sure.

We made certain to include her in the marriage ceremony by presenting her a locket with a photo of her mom on one side and a photo of Terri on the other. She broke down crying. In time she came to accept Terri completely. After all, Terri was far more hip in her music tastes and a much better cook. We became a family in short order.

Although battered and bruised by her learning difficulties over the years, even in her studies Jessica had made steady progress in her final two years in high school. I felt proud of how far she'd come and made sure to tell her so.

As Jessica's graduation approached, Terri and I devoted time in the hospital toward planning a celebration for her. By now, I'd completed my downhill slide from cane to walker to hospital, soon to come home in a wheelchair. There was no longer any denying the seriousness of my condition, and Jessica had taken pride in caring for me over the past months in any way she could. Despite her learning disabilities, she had good social instincts. She was sensitive and kind, a "people person" as we sometimes called her. She had an uncanny ability to size up the motives of adults as well as her peers in things of importance. While math and verbal studies baffled her, nothing in the realm of social interaction escaped her antennae. Although frightened by my deteriorating condition, she felt some relief as I stabilized, and as Terri and I finally came to accept the reality of our new world order.

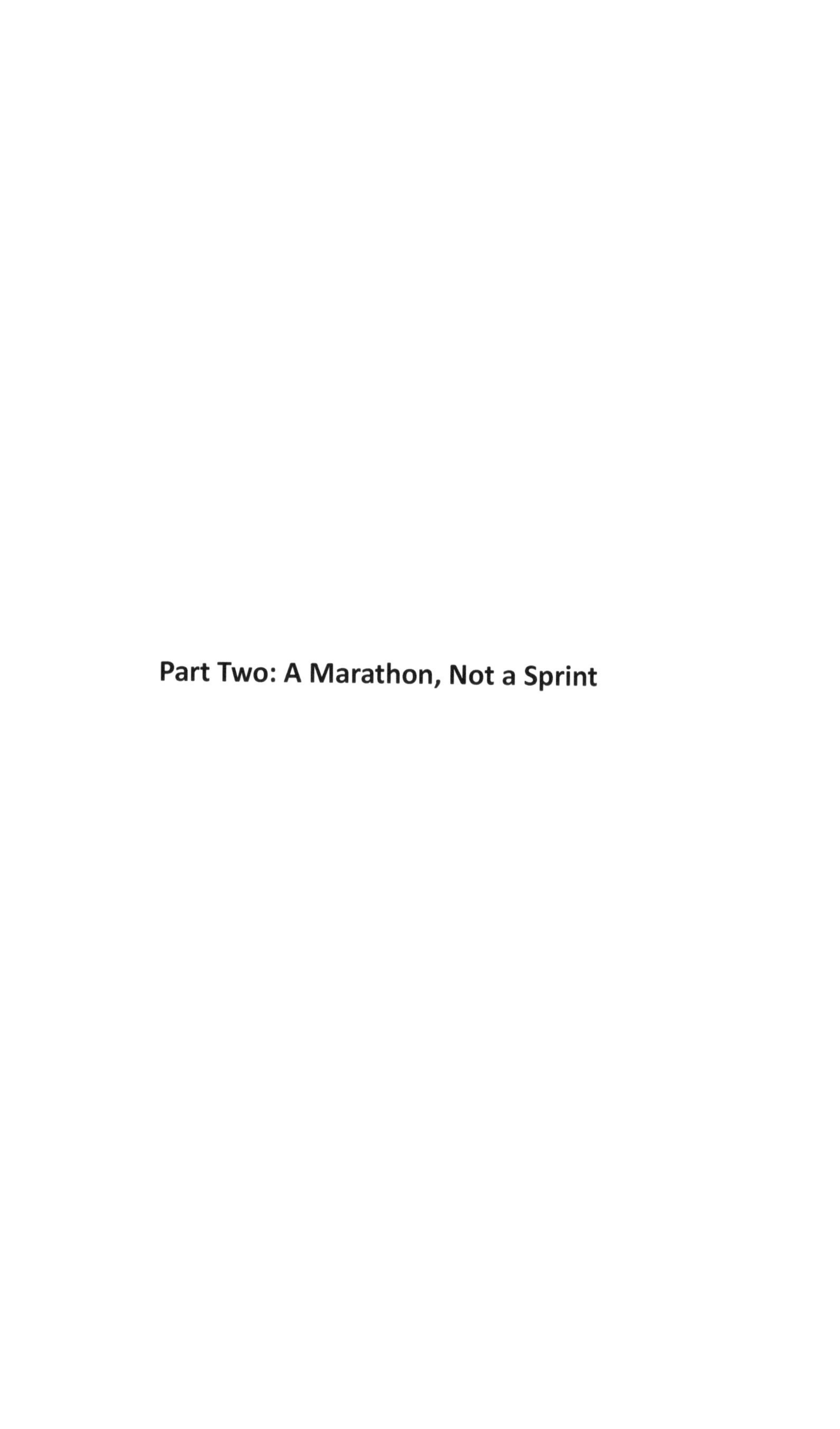

Part Two: A Marathon, Not a Sprint

8 My New World Order

Following the first physical therapy session early in my hospital adventure, little time elapsed before a knock on my half-opened door awakened me from my daydreaming. “Come in,” I said without much enthusiasm. Michelle, my assigned occupational therapist, entered bringing along a young trainee named Judith. “A hospital is no place to rest,” I muttered to myself.

Physical therapists work with patients to improve the strength of muscles and physical activities like walking and balance. Michelle and Judith, as occupational therapists, focused on improving or compensating for deficiency in fine motor skills, particularly the use of fingers, hands and arms, to complete basic tasks.

Michelle, a short woman in her early thirties with short-cut brown hair, casually dressed in jeans and a sweater, came bearing gifts: an array of toys and gadgets in a large red sack. The red sack reminded me of Christmas mornings when I, with my older cousins, snuck downstairs in our family’s summer home on the Jersey shore, where we spent winter breaks, to find that the 12-foot high Christmas tree had been magically decorated overnight. Surrounding the tree were exquisitely wrapped gifts and stockings for each of us. With gleeful anticipation, we tackled our stockings, pulling out little surprises one by one, keeping painfully quiet so as not to awaken the adults who were sleeping off the effects of a rollicking Christmas Eve party. We knew we couldn't unwrap the gifts until after breakfast.

In my stocking I might find a car or two from the Matchbox series to add to my collection. I'd hope for a Studebaker or yellow school bus. Or, I might find a tightly rolled up monster magazine, possibly an edition of *Famous Monsters of Filmland*. I'd become addicted to old monster movies such as *Dracula* or *The Werewolf of London*. Bela Lugosi was my favorite film star, my absolute favorite, even more so than Doris Day on whom I nursed a schoolboy crush. Also in my stocking, there might be a small puzzle or game of some sort that required Patsy or Judy to show me how it worked. At the bottom of the stocking would be an apple or banana.

This hospital setting, however, was not fun and the gifts were anything but playthings. Michelle and Judith, a tall, attractive black woman in her mid-twenties, pulled up chairs as I sat up on the side of my bed. Michelle spoke first as Judith, interning as a graduate student, listened carefully.

Michelle explained the benefits of occupational therapy, letting me know that I'd be spending these sessions with them lifting light weights, putting pegs in holes, and performing more functional chores, such as testing my way around a makeshift kitchen. "I've studied the hospital notes about you," she said as she reached back for the sack, "but you tell us what are your main concerns."

How could I begin to convey the helplessness I felt, the suffocating fear that I'd never get better. "Everything," I said. "I have no use of my fingers and my wrists are weak. I can't dress myself without help. Socks, shoes and buttons are impossible. I can't bend down or reach up for things. I can't unlock the door to my apartment or turn a key."

"We brought some stuff that may be of use to you," she said, as she opened the sack containing a variety of gizmos. First she pulled out a large blue key holder. "This should help with using keys," she said as she inserted one of her own keys into the holder. "A large extension like this will allow you to open any door simply by turning it with your hand. The key locks in and turns with the holder. " This I would find useful as the absence of finger muscles made it impossible for me to maneuver any kind of key without an attachment that I could grip with my hand.

Then they introduced me to an object that, for lack of a better name, I will call a grabber stick. By squeezing the handle on top of the stick, the claw at the bottom would open, allowing me to pick up items from the floor or reach for objects up high. Michelle took a Kleenex from my bedside table and let it fall on the floor in front of me. "See if you can grab the tissue with the grabber," she said, handing me the implement. I couldn't squeeze the handle with one hand, but by using both hands I could apply enough force to retrieve the Kleenex. In the days ahead I'd find that my fingers and wrists were too weak to squeeze hard enough to grab anything of any size, especially from kitchen cabinets up high, although I could make limited use of it to reach items on the floor, like a magazine or paperback book. I'd reach for the item with the stick, drag it back within easy reach, squeeze the handle with both hands, and voila, success. "You keep this near you and practice," said Michelle. Judith took it from me and leaned it against the wall by my bed.

Next came a so-called buttonhook that, if I worked it right, could allow me to button and unbutton my shirts or pants compensating for my lack of finger dexterity. Michelle demonstrated by hooking a button on my polo shirt and maneuvering the button through the button slit. "Now you try," she said.

I fumbled with it for several minutes. I could get the small hook around the button, but as soon as I attempted to maneuver it through the slit, the button slipped off the hook and I had to start again from scratch. I withheld the urge to swear. "Let me try it with the button open," I said. I spent the next few minutes trying to get my button closed again, but to no avail. "It's easier to just buy polo shirts with only one button on top that I could leave open," I said.

"That is certainly one option," Michelle agreed, "but let's try again later." Michelle was not ready to let me off the hook—or buttonhook—so soon.

In the coming weeks, in order to alleviate the frustration

of getting dressed, Terri found a company in California that specialized in clothes for mobility-impaired folks like me. She ordered several pairs of pants with Velcro straps in lieu of buttons or belt loops. In the meantime, I banished the buttonhook to a drawer, where it remained throughout my occupational therapy.

Of all the gadgets that Michelle and Judith presented to me, the most ingenious was an object that, if I could master it, would allow me to put socks on without bending down or pulling my legs up. I could fold my socks around a plastic holder, and then place my feet a certain way, and the socks would magically unfold onto my feet. Here again, the weakness of my grip and lack of finger movement made this thingamajig too difficult for me to manipulate. But I thought it quite an invention. I accepted a two-foot-long shoehorn instead. I might at least be able to make use of that.

Toward the end of the hour, Michelle tested my hand, wrist and arm muscles, as Judith looked on. My wrists didn't work at all against gravity. Whenever I lifted my arm above my head as if to wave to someone, my hand drooped down like a dying tulip. My fingers displayed even less mobility.

"Try moving your fingers apart one at a time," Michelle instructed. Not much luck. I could barely separate them. "Now try touching each of your four fingers with your thumb," she said. Less success. I couldn't even make the universal obscene gesture with my middle finger. I dreamed of the day when I could once again master this feat. I imagined that I would show off my newfound dexterity to Dr. Richardson, saying, "Look, look doctor, I can drive again."

I knew that I'd have to master basic tasks through occupational therapy, but having to learn from scratch brought back painful memories of hardships I'd encountered in my past in performing tasks with my hands, a certain clumsiness I'd had as a kid doing even simple things like tying a tie, devising a knot, or stringing lights on a Christmas tree. To make matters worse my cousins used to mock me for lacking manual dexterity.

Also, patience was never my strong suit. I'd get frustrated easily if I had to figure out how to do something new. I'd developed something of a mental block about fixing or repairing things that most people had little trouble with, like changing a spare tire. I'd prefer buying furniture already assembled rather than something I'd have to put together myself. I'd gotten over that to some extent, but now I'd have to learn altogether new tricks and strategies to survive on my own. I wasn't mentally prepared for this new world order.

With physical therapy I could sense that persistence in exercising or lifting weights (plain old hard work) would lead to improvement in my condition over time. But it struck me that by using gadgets to help dress myself or navigate my way around my own kitchen was tantamount to a resignation of sorts that I was now helpless and might be for the rest of my life. None of this was true, of course. These tricks were simply ways to help me get by each day until I got better. But I felt defeated and drained of the energy necessary to make the effort. I submitted to the routine anyway. Doing so was my only recourse if I wanted to cope. "It's temporary," I kept telling myself. And some of the games were fun, like seeing how fast I could remove pegs from holes on a board and then put them back. Maybe on this day or that I'd set a personal record. In this way my competitive spirit prevailed. In any event, it might make me a little more independent. Who was I to say otherwise?

Michelle devised an agenda for me for the coming sessions. Judith appeared alone the next couple of days, but she didn't really know her stuff well enough to answer my questions or to suggest alternative strategies when I became frustrated. She was pleasant enough to work with and deferential to my wants. Too deferential. What I needed was a good kick in the pants. I mentioned to Michelle that I felt I needed to be in the hands of a more experienced therapist. Michelle seemed to understand. She was older and more experienced than Judith and had a better sense of what I was willing or able to do. From then on, she worked alone with me every day.

When Michelle and Judith had finished their first session with me that day, it was close to 5 o'clock. Terri would arrive in a couple of hours. We'd agreed she would bring pizza so we could dine together at the hospital. So when dinner was brought I refused it, telling the attendant defiantly that I'd be dining on pizza shortly.

"Lucky you," she said. In the next moment I was dozing.

At seven or so, Terri came in, balancing her rolling brief case in one hand and the pizza in the other. "Hi, sweetie pie," she said.

"I'm so glad to see you. I've missed you all day," I said.

"I've missed you too, and look, I brought the mail. We can open it and do bills after dinner." She knew I wanted to keep up with the daily routine, albeit with her help. "Let's eat first though."

It pleased me to hear she'd gotten the pizza at Luigi's. We'd never been there together, but she knew how fond I was of Luigi's pizza as I'd talked about it enough.

"Well now I'm famished. Did you bring the merlot?"

"Now, now, you know that's contraband here. You'll have to make do with Diet Coke or Sprite. You pick."

Munching on the pizza, I told her about my day, venting my frustration with the OT session. "It was like trying to learn how to tie a knot," I said. Terri chuckled as she reached for a second slice of pizza. She knew the tall story I liked to tell: that my mother wanted me to join the Navy and sail to faraway lands, but since I couldn't do knots, I ran away from home and went to law school instead. "Maybe I'll sign up with the Army tomorrow," I said.

"You'd have a hard time firing a gun, squeezing the trigger."

"I'm sure Michelle could devise some sort of attachment." We both laughed.

When we finished eating, Terri raised the bed and helped me get up and settle in the one large vinyl armchair in my otherwise spartan room. The other bed was empty for the time being, my roommate having been released the day before. We knew this privacy would be short-lived. When I was comfortably seated, Terri came over and hugged me.

"I don't know why this is happening to you. What I do know is that we will get through it together and you will get better," she said.

"You'll stay with me, no matter what?

"We're in this together. You've treated me like a queen. We will be fine."

"Always?" I asked.

"Always. What's important is that you're still who you are. You've still got your mind. Just think how hard it would be if you had Alzheimer's or something that affected you mentally. We'll deal with this together, you and me, as we do everything. We'll get through this." She hugged me tight as she was speaking.

"But how will I do everything I used to do?" I ticked off a list. Helping with dinner parties, groceries, all sorts of errands, driving. "You know how much you hate to drive."

"Listen, we can do all that together. Yeah, I'm not crazy about driving, but I'll do it until you get better. And you *will* get better." She reassured me that I'd be able to return to work before long, that the social worker had ordered a motorized chair and our insurance would cover it. "Thank goodness for your job and health benefits. And just think, if you had a physical job and couldn't work at all, how hard that would be. Things could be a whole lot worse. Oh, and next week I'll bring your driver's license to the MVA—I think it's at Sixth and E—with the medical letters to apply for a handicap placard."

She also assured me that if I was well enough to drive by November, I could turn the placard in and get my license back. "The office has put in for a space in the Marriott garage next door. That'll make going to and from work really easy, especially since we work in the same building."

She was speaking quickly, too quickly, and when I looked into her eyes, I saw they were glistening with tears.

Of course, I knew she'd never leave me, no matter what. She'd often reminded me that in the years since we met her life had gotten so much better. She suffered from a guilt complex that most likely was a product of her parents' contentious divorce during her college years. Her mom Eleanor, a bright but emotionally volatile woman, never got over the divorce and spent much of her days working on a project aimed at getting even with her ex-husband, who she referred to as "that bastard." Terri was caught in the middle.

When we met in 1997, Terri had just started her job as a

lawyer with the Justice Department. She'd given up her job at a prestigious law firm, a position she'd taken out of concern that she'd soon be called upon to support her mother, who had difficulty holding down jobs. Working with a particularly nasty partner made her time at the firm stressful. That, in addition to coping with her mother's persistent disregard for social boundaries, proved too much for her to handle. She soon landed in the hospital for depression.

Eleanor's difficulty respecting boundaries was no small thing. Terri shared the townhouse she owned in a Maryland suburb with two other women. Her mom, who lived too close for comfort, would frequently come over to Terri's house without invitation or notice, sometimes with the intent to re-arrange the furniture or plant trees in the front yard. When Terri was admitted to the hospital, Eleanor brooded that her daughter would miss Eleanor's performance in a local production of *Macbeth*. She solved this dilemma by performing a particularly gruesome scene from *Macbeth* in the hospital reception room for an audience of Terri and a handful of other patients, which worked until the nurses ushered her out. Eleanor was incensed when Terri's doctors banned her from future unsupervised visits.

Terri insisted that I'd saved her by providing her with a healthier perspective on how to deal with her family. Perhaps now would be the opportunity to return the favor. I wasn't so sure, however, that this would turn out to be a fair exchange. "When this is over and I'm all better I'll make this up to you, big time. I love you so much," I said. "Your being here has already cheered me up." She hugged me tight and cried softly.

After a while, she took a deep breath and I knew she was better. We looked over the mail, paid some bills, and then watched CNN. Keeping to as close a normal routine as possible lifted my spirits in a way that neither Zoloft nor any other medicine could ever do. I resolved to return to the office as soon as I could. I wasn't about to put my life on hold.

Around nine o'clock, the announcement came that visiting hours were over, an edict that we ignored and would continue to ignore. No one seemed inclined to bother us about it.

By ten o'clock, it was time for Terri to go home. She made certain I had what I needed on the table next to me, including my toothbrush, toothpaste and rinse bowl for the morning. She brushed my teeth with my electric brush, pulled my sheets up, and then hugged me good night.

"Good night, I love you sweetheart."

"I love you too," I said. "I can't wait until you come again tomorrow. I'll call you in the morning."

I felt one hundred thousand times better from Terri's visit. How could I go through this alone? I was also extremely sleepy. The last two days had seemed an eternity. I put my head back against the pillow and closed my eyes.

As busy as the last couple of days in the hospital had been, the nighttime activity didn't let up. The woman down the hall who had wailed throughout the previous night was at it again with a vengeance. She was moaning and hollering as if she was being beaten and whipped by a dozen or more wicked nurses. I called for a nurse to come shut my door. After that came a knock on my door. The nurse's aide on night duty came in rolling in her cart ready to take my temperature and blood pressure.

"You just did that a couple of hours ago," I said.

"That's right, you're on a two-hour schedule for temperature and blood pressure."

We accomplished both tasks quickly. I was too sleepy to complain. As she left, she and her cart became a blur to me.

All of a sudden I'm outdoors and start making my way toward a crowd of people. They're gathered for a road race, probably a 10k. I begin jogging and soon I join a group of folks I know, friends from college or law school. I see a colleague from my office. "Look at me, I can run too now," I say. Then I find myself jogging uphill along a familiar route. I circle around a fountain and head back downhill, winding up at a gym where I'd left my hospital gown.

The nurse's aide appears again, this time in the gym. I hold out my arm for my blood pressure to be taken while keeping the thermometer securely under my tongue. Then I'm running along a riverbank that resembles a bayou in Louisiana. An alligator is resting on the opposite bank. He poses no imminent threat. I pick up the pace and soon I'm running at a fast, steady clip, mindful of the creatures that could pop out at me at any time, from the tree branches above, the forest to my left, or the slimy green water along my right. I run a long, long way always looking around me.

I hear a knock on my door. I sit up, nearly awake.

It was the morning nurse's aide who waltzed right in without awaiting an invitation. "Time to wash up."

I yawned. It must be morning. The clock on the wall told me it was five o'clock. I'd slept pretty well, just not long enough. A hospital is no place to come for a rest, I thought again.

"Would you like me to help you wash?"

"As soon as I have a chance to brush my teeth," I said.

"Okay, I'll come back shortly." She left and when I had brushed my teeth I sat up to see whether I could stand up. The bed was too low. I could only stand if the bed was cranked up to a sufficient height. If it was high enough, I could just pop up onto my feet. What worried me more was that my hands seemed to be getting weaker still. At ten o'clock I would have my first of a series of plasmapheresis treatments where I'd be hooked to a machine that separated blood from plasma in the hopes of tricking my immune system into ceasing its attack on my peripheral nerves. I was skeptical, as nothing else had worked so far. Something had better work soon.

Eighteen months: it seemed like a long time to wait, but it also dawned on me that it might be too short a spell. What if my nerves needed longer to re-generate? What then?

9 A Marathon, Not A Sprint

There was no therapy on Sundays, but lots of visitors to divert my thoughts away from self-pity and keep my frustration in check. With Easter coming up the following week, more than two weeks into my hospital stay, I could tell Terri and Jane were planning something, but I wasn't sure what. I knew just enough to understand that I'd have to dress in more formal attire than pajamas. "Be dressed and ready by noon," Terri warned me the day before. "You'll have visitors."

"Who?" I asked.

"You'll see," was all she let on.

Around two in the afternoon on Easter Sunday I could hear chatter in the corridor outside my room.

"Who's got the plates and silverware?"

"I've got the lamb. And here's the mint sauce. Terri has the plates."

"I have the silverware and napkins."

These were the voices of friends and co-workers. Jane led the charge, and I could hear Gay and now Sheila. It was Easter Sunday and my friends had talked my wife into celebrating Easter with us at the hospital. I was now in the rehab unit that had a nicely appointed dining room. It had half a dozen tables of varying sizes, a blue wall-to-wall carpet, a fish tank, and a cabinet with books and games. Best of all, the room was generally vacant during the hours between lunch and dinner. My guests began to speak in hushed voices and tiptoed directly to the dining room—this was supposed to be a surprise after all—where they started laying out a table for a festive dinner with table cloth, candles, silverware, real plates, cloth napkins, the whole shebang.

I hope they keep it quiet, I thought to myself, so no one will mind us. Ah, that would be asking too much of this group.

After everything had been set up, Terri came to get me. "I don't need the chair," I said. "Let me walk in." She brought my walker and accompanied me down the hall and into the dining room. I wanted to show that I still had some of the old mobility left. I proudly approached the table to the applause and cheers of our small crowd.

Jane, no doubt, had spearheaded this pleasant surprise. She and Terri had remained mum about it, although I bet it was in the planning for a week or more. Gay, who was about my age, had worked in the same office as me for many years; in fact, her office was next door to mine. Often, in mid-afternoon we'd stroll over to Starbucks for coffee to help us get through the day. Sheila, a couple of years my elder, had been a co-worker when I had first started at Justice's Civil Rights Division in the early 70's. She and Gay became golfing buddies after meeting one another at my wedding to Terri a few years back.

Jane's Foreign Service experience had helped make her adept in the art of arranging dinner parties. The candles were lit and a colorful arrangement of flowers, borrowed from my hospital room, served as a centerpiece. Lamb, roast potatoes, asparagus, salad, rolls, and more were placed on the table. Terri sat beside me so she could help serve me food and cut my meat. Gay poured the wine, while Jane dished out generous portions of each dish onto my plate. What a delightful departure from hospital food.

"I'd like a glass of wine too," I said.

"Terri?" Jane looked to my wife for a green light to allow me the wine.

"Well. I suppose one glass won't hurt."

Now I was in heaven. "Where are the musicians?" I teased.

"You mean you can't hear them." Everyone laughed. An old

lady, a patient from down the hall, was singing loudly to herself.

"Oops, we forgot the jelly," Gay said. "Ah, here it is. Would you like some mint jelly for the lamb, Michael?"

"Sure." She passed it to me. "Wait a minute. This jelly isn't mint, it's jalapeno. How rascally of you." Everyone knew about my taste for spicy food. No detail was overlooked in their endeavor to please and tease me.

As far back as I remember, I've been addicted to hot spicy food, the zing of the heat on the tip of my tongue, spreading to the sides of my mouth, to the back of my throat, beads of sweat forming on my brow, fire flaring from my mouth like Godzilla. Pure heaven. However, my affection for culinary heat has at times gotten me in trouble. I recall such a time with mild regret.

It was Thanksgiving, 1981—a few months after Jessica was born—when my wife Sylvia and I invited my quirky relatives to our home in D.C. to have their first look at the baby. I wanted to make something different. Sylvia had cooked a tasty chicken mole once, not too spicy in my judgment, though my judgment was skewed, like the taste buds on my tongue, seared to oblivion by countless encounters with hot chili peppers. Because it was Thanksgiving, it seemed appropriate to shift the recipe to turkey. I retain the following vision of how this sorrowful event unfolded.

Sylvia and I are in the kitchen the weekend before, she nursing Jessica while I'm fixing a salad for dinner. "If your mother, Aunt Ceal, Uncle Lou, Patsy and Judy all come you'll need to book three rooms," Sylvia says. "And what will you make?"

"I was thinking turkey mole, just to be creative," I say.

"Don't Sis and Lou have ulcers?" Sylvia asks.

"It won't be too spicy, trust me," I say.

"Okay, it's your family."

The following evening, I combine the ingredients according to the recipe, except I realize too late that I forgot to remove the seeds from the chilies. No matter, there's still time for the spices to blend, making for a fine sauce. Anyway, ancho and poblano chilies are relatively mild as hot chilies go.

The gang arrives Thursday in their customary style like a runaway train caught in a tornado. Patsy rushes in first. "Hi

Mikey, hello Syl, how are you? Where's the baby? Oh there, how adorable. I've got to use the bathroom. Where can I put this?" She removes her fur coat. "Never mind, I'll just throw it here." She drapes it around the banister. Judy peeks at the baby as she puffs on her cigarette.

"Boy it's cold in here," Ceal says, shivering. Sylvia explains that the furnace conked out that morning. Ceal and Sis, their orange bouffants recently freshened, hover together keeping on their coats, and proceed to light up. Lou joins them saying little.

Following cocktails, Sylvia ushers everyone into the dining room and then takes her place, nursing the baby. Salad finished, she puts Jessica in the bassinet and goes to fetch the mole. Ceal turns to me, and says in a hushed voice, "What's she doing? Nursing the baby at the table? I never heard of such a thing."

"Oh, it's normal these days," I explain, "And look, here comes the mole."

Ceal takes a bite. I hold my breath. "It's awfully spicy," she rasps. Then Lou shovels a heaping into his mouth. I cringe as he jolts back from the table.

"I can't eat this shit, Ceal. Make me a scrambled egg."

Ceal leans over to me, "Michael, you know Sis and Lou have ulcers."

"I'll make eggs," Sylvia says, glaring at me. I follow Sylvia into the kitchen. "Trust you," she says. "What a dumb idea, and your family is so rude. They never asked once about me or Jessica. They are the most self-absorbed people on the planet. And if Patsy calls me Syl one more time, I'll throw the mole sauce in her face."

Sylvia brings the eggs to the table. "Pass the so called tortillas," my mother says.

Luckily, I didn't create the menu for this Easter feast. The aroma from the lamb and hot rolls cast out the antiseptic odors that pervaded the corridors of the hospital. Now I was transported to a fine restaurant. For a few hours I forgot about my disability and the struggles that lay ahead. I just enjoyed the companionship of a few close friends, as well as the care taken in the preparation of the food and the table. I can get through this, I thought, with the support of my wife and family and friends.

In between courses, I reminisced with Sheila about old acquaintances from our days in Civil Rights. Sheila still worked there, albeit in a different section than the one in which we had worked together.

I had come of age in the era when news screens were dominated by southern church bombings, lunch counter protests, dogs attacking marchers, and water hoses unleashed on black citizens by the likes of Sheriff Clark and his boys. I was captivated and appalled by these events. In college in Ohio, I studied American History, concentrating on the old south, slavery, and the Civil War period. While attending law school in Washington, I took part in the protests against the war in Vietnam. And I took a keen interest in civil liberties issues. So, in the fall of 1973, following a one-year clerkship for a federal judge in New York, I eagerly accepted an offer of employment as trial attorney in the Civil Rights Division at Justice. If I could lend a hand, however small, to the cause of equal justice, I might feel fulfilled in my chosen profession.

With my return to Washington (and hopefully not because of it) it seemed that the Justice Department, and, indeed, the entire government was on the verge of collapse. During my first week on the job, the Attorney General, Eliot Richardson, was forced to resign because he refused to follow President Nixon's order to fire Archibald Cox, the Watergate special prosecutor. Richardson's second-in-command also resigned and it was left to Robert Bork, then the Solicitor General, to fire Cox, which he dutifully did. As history buffs no doubt recall, these events became known as the "Saturday Night Massacre." Some of my colleagues and I walked the three blocks from our office to the Great Hall at the Main Justice building to listen to Richardson's resignation speech. Our Section Chief held a meeting that afternoon to assure us that we were still in business. Soon after, Congress began impeachment proceedings: an ominous start to my legal career.

Sheila and I had shared other compelling moments in Civil Rights. One of our first travel assignments was to conduct a pre-election survey in Wilcox County, Alabama. The purpose of the survey was to determine the need for sending federal observers to cover the upcoming primary elections there. The prospect of this trip, my first foray into the Deep South, filled me with a sense of foreboding.

Wilcox County, I knew, was in the heart of Alabama's black belt, a region so named for the richness of its soil rather than for its majority African American population. Wilcox, Dallas, Lowndes, Hale, Greene Counties: all landmarks of the tumultuous 60's. "Wilcox County is all backwoods and forest," one of the more seasoned lawyers told me. "There's one town, Camden, the county seat. You'll have an awful time among the unmarked dirt roads just finding the polling places."

I understood that we'd stay in Selma, about 40 miles north, our best option. Monroeville, where *To Kill A Mockingbird* was filmed, was just 40 miles down the highway from Camden. "We'll speak to Reverend Threadgill first," Sheila suggested as we started to discuss our plan of action. "He knows everything that goes on in the county. Then we'll be armed with enough information to interview the election officials."

The time for going to Alabama came fast enough. It was dark as we made the drive from Montgomery to Selma. If only the trees could speak. They had borne vivid witness to the marches, the singing, the beatings and killings that had taken place along this route a decade earlier. I was in high school in Manhattan then. I never thought that I would actually travel here, to the Deep South, to Alabama, to help further the cause. True, things had changed dramatically since the 60's, but I was nevertheless thrilled to be able to speak with the folks who had lived through and witnessed all these things.

The next day we spoke to Rev. Threadgill. I won't vouch for the names of all of the people and places, but the conversation went something like this:

"We glad to see you folks. Trouble is brewing," the reverend said.

"What trouble specifically, Reverend?"

"They kicked out our poll watchers over in Sardis. They up to no good. Stole votes in Sardis last time."

"Where do they vote in Sardis?"

"In Mrs. Ames' antique store."

"Where is that exactly?"

"Take the Samsonville road until you see a gas station/general store. Turn down the dirt road there, make your first left."

"Onto another dirt road?" I asked.

"That's the only roads there is in those parts."

"Okay," I said. "Then what?"

"Go down that road a piece and you see her store on the right. Her mutts are all around the store. Can't miss it."

After meeting with Rev. Threadgill, we went to the courthouse in Camden to speak to the probate judge. In Alabama, the county probate judge ran the elections. She greeted us like old friends. "Well now, if it isn't the federal boys. How you doing boys?" Her attitude appeared shrewd and polished, marked by a pretense of good humor and seasoned by years of dealing with federal workers from Washington. "We've no problems here in Wilcox County. People get along real well. Y'all are most welcome to watch all you like."

Without feeling terribly reassured, we went on to interview a few more people and then returned to Selma. "Oops, we forgot to call the office," Sheila reminded me. Probably as a consequence of the hostility of the previous decade, the office maintained a policy of requiring its lawyers to call in twice a day (more often during election coverage) to report on the day's events, or lack thereof. I was admonished on occasion for missing a call. ("Gee, I got wrapped up in so many interviews all morning, I just forgot").

The next morning we drove out to Sardis to speak with Mrs. Ames. At first I didn't see anyone, so I walked to the back of the store. There, in the rear, I saw a wizened old white lady sweeping the floor. I assumed that this woman was Mrs. Ames. No sooner did I start to question her regarding the complaints about lost ballots, when she came toward me waving her broom. Was she going to swing it at me or was this only her attempt at intimidation? She shouted at me in her high-pitched voice.

"I'm sick and tired of you people nosing into our business. We never had no trouble out here 'til the niggers started voting."

I'm not sure whether Sheila or I drafted the report on the plane ride home, but I'm confident that we recommended that federal observers be sent to Wilcox County for the primary election that year.

I returned to Alabama and other states in the south many times during my six plus years with Civil Rights. During the 60's the primary mission of the Civil Rights Division had been voter registration. Under the Voting Rights Act of 1965, federal examiners were sent into the South to register voters, so by the time Sheila and I came along this mission was largely accomplished. State and local election officials in black belt counties had turned instead to more subtle means of discrimination. We initiated lawsuits to assure that black voters, who'd been victims of discrimination in the past, were given an equal opportunity to elect candidates of their choice.

One such case involved Hale County, Alabama. I needed witnesses to testify to the lingering effect of past discriminatory practices to justify imposition of single member districts. Witnesses were hard to find because many older blacks were afraid to ask their white employees for time off for anything. As a black lawyer from Selma explained to me, the plantation mentality still had a firm hold, especially on the elderly, in rural black belt counties.

By luck, I found a woman named Theresa who had been active in registering voters in the 60's. She was waiting for me on the front porch of her single story wood-frame house as I drove up in my rental car. We sat outside as her air conditioner was on the fritz and it was brutally hot and musty inside. She served us her homemade brew of sweet tea. I wasted no time asking her to tell me about her efforts to register voters in the days preceding passage of the Voting Rights Act. She told me this story as if it had happened only a day ago:

There was this minister who's now deceased and he and I would go to the courthouse together and we'd attempt to register. We'd ask for the form, and they'd be sitting playing dominoes around the table, all of them would be sitting around, and we would stand

and wait while they played dominoes. And then they would say "Well what you want, girl," or "What is it gal? What are you up here for?" And we'd say, "we came to register," and they would continue to play, and we'd continue to stand. Maybe it would take two hours, maybe one, maybe three that we would stand there. And they would play dominoes.

Theresa pauses and we each take a sip of ice tea. Go on, I say. This is just what I need to hear. She continues:

And, so finally they would take a paper and throw it to us and say, "write the second line of the second paragraph or the first line of the Constitution," something of that sort along with your name, your age, your address, and why you want to vote. All this—these are the types of forms they had for us to fill out.

Theresa tells the story so well I resolve to ask her to repeat it when I take her deposition to use at trial that will be held in Washington, D.C.

We won the Hale County case and best of all, the Court repeated Theresa's story *verbatim* in its factual findings.

Despite frustration with bureaucracy, and seemingly endless review of memos and court filings, my experience in Civil Rights was rewarding. Luckily, I moved on before the Reagan administration did its best to restrain vigorous enforcement of civil rights laws. Sheila remained at Civil Rights for more than 30 years. I admire her perseverance, as well as the perseverance of those activists in the civil rights movement who fought so hard for so long for what is right.

Perseverance. I needed some of that now.

We ate the almond raspberry cake that Gay had brought and drank a little more of the sparkling wine. Then, we chatted a while, taking advantage of our little oasis in the hospital. By mid-afternoon it was time to clean up. I thanked Sheila, Jane, and Gay for the surprise Easter dinner and wished them good-bye. Then I shuffled back down the hall to my room. Terri left for a while to browse through CDs at Tower Records, just two blocks away.

I lay back on my bed to rest. For the first time in a long while I was feeling cheerful and relaxed.

It was a day or two after Easter Sunday. I lay on my bed feeling dozy after the last therapy session of the day. Soon, Terri would arrive with a few of her relatives, including Uncle Howard, a doctor. I gazed sleepily at the scores of get-well cards, plants and flowers that adorned my windowsill. But the high that I had experienced just a couple of days before was spiraling downward. Just as my spirits rose to the fun of the Easter festivities, they now plunged like mountaineers swept off a precarious ledge in a furious storm, as thoughts of the enormity of my handicap and the uncertainty of any recovery overcame me. How can I continue to do even the most mundane tasks of my daily life? Isn't it too much to ask of my wife, daughter, and friends to help me function in the most basic things of life, day after day after day? What if I don't recover? There are no guarantees. What if in 18 months I am just like today, needing help simply getting out of a chair, or getting dressed, or cutting my food, or taking a shower? Even if I can go back to work with the help of a motorized chair, I still won't be able to travel anywhere without Terri. No colleague can help me with my personal needs. I can't even drive anymore.

As these thoughts plagued me, Terri walked in, accompanied by her uncle Howard, his wife Judy, and her Aunt Julia, who had driven down from New York. I'd known they would be coming so I'd put on pajamas and a robe instead of the skimpy hospital gown. I wasn't much in the mood for a family visit, but I welcomed everyone nonetheless. Julia seemed aghast at my emaciated appearance. After some introductory small talk, Howard said he wanted to speak privately to me. The women excused themselves saying they would go for coffee.

Howard is a medical doctor who had suffered from a rare and debilitating neurological illness triggered by an automobile accident. He had since partially recovered, but he still wore a neck brace due to painful back and neck spasms. To his great frustration, the medical profession knew of no cure or treatment for his condition. Prior to his illness, he had practiced gastroenterology, performing all of the medical procedures related to his field. However, his illness, which caused him unrelenting pain, had forced him to relinquish this practice. He'd refused to give up though. While he could no longer perform medical procedures, he'd turned his medical career around to become one of the foremost experts in pain management, providing advice to medical practitioners and government agencies, while flying all over the globe to lecture on various aspects of his newly developed specialty.

"You seem to be coping well," he said to me.

"Well, I have a lot of support," I said. "Especially from Terri, but also my friends and my office have been great. Most importantly, the prognosis is that I'll recover. I just hope that it starts to happen soon."

"Just keep in mind that neurological recovery is painfully slow," Howard said. "You won't see improvement day to day, or even week to week. You may see that you can use your hands or arms a little better each month. The touchstone here is patience. I've spoken to your doctors as I promised. You are in a marathon, not a sprint." Howard knew the running metaphor would be something I could relate to.

"I suppose so," I said, not particularly pleased with the message. Resigned to its wisdom, perhaps. But not pleased.

"The important thing for you," he continued, "just as it was with me, is that you are who you are. No one can take away your resolve, your competitiveness, your spirit. Your body may be broken for now, but your mind remains strong. I had a lot of anger when I was stricken. One time, when some dumb fuck parked illegally in a handicap space, I slashed the tires on his car. I know it was a foolish thing to do, and Judy told me so, but I was angry at the world. The most meaningful thing was that Judy stood by me one hundred percent the whole time. Some people would ask her how could you stay with him? She'll tell you that. She stood with me just as Terri is one hundred percent behind you."

"I couldn't do this without her," I said.

"And how is Jessica doing?"

"She's been great too. She may have learning disabilities, but she has great people instincts. She likes to help me in any way she can.

"That's great. My sons, of course, were a lot younger than your daughter. When I was wheelchair-bound they would challenge my authority in various ways. Judy and I put a stop to that."

"That isn't an issue with Jess," I said. "I think she responds especially well to my vulnerability. She's a sensitive girl."

I thought of the time when, shortly before her death, my mother had been moved to a nursing home in Chevy Chase, wheelchair-bound and suffering from severe dementia. We'd drive up to visit several times a week taking chocolates, since she was no longer allowed to smoke. At dinner, Jessica would sit right next to her in order to ensure that she ate at least some of her unappealing plate of ground up meat and soggy vegetables. "Grandma, just one bite," Jessica would insist, time and again. So patient. So caring.

"Let me ask you this," Howard said, changing the topic. "Do you have much pain?"

"Luckily, I don't have much pain," I said, "even though many patients with CIDP do have pain. I have this strange buzzing in my feet that comes and goes. Mostly, my feet are stiff and numb, although it hurts like hell if I bang them on the footboard. These hospital beds are way too short."

"How do your hands feel?"

"Prickly, like pins and needles, but they don't really hurt. It's hard to describe."

"It's a blessing that you've dodged that bullet. I was—still am—in pain. Which explains why I'm now doing what I'm doing."

I told Howard what Dr. Richardson said about having 18 months for the nerves to regenerate before muscle wasting occurs, and also that CIDP patients who recover usually do so within a year. Howard then explained that it all depended on the extent of nerve damage and whether some nerves had been severed.

"It's really impossible to predict your outcome now. Just remember, you are running a marathon here. This is not a sprint." Howard would repeat these words often in the long and difficult weeks and months ahead.

The women returned and after visiting for a while, Howard, Judy, and Julia said goodbye and wished me well. Terri stayed with me for the evening. I told her what Howard had said, especially the part about this being a marathon.

"How am I going to play my part—do all the things that we've divided up?" I moaned. "Watering the plants, taking out the garbage, doing the dishes, helping with the cooking, getting dressed and showered? It stinks, I can't do anything useful."

"For God's sake, Michael, I didn't marry you so you could take out the garbage. Howard is exactly right that you're the same person you always were. You are smart and resilient and competitive, my very best friend. Someone I can always trust. Some people would give up and fall to pieces but that's not who you are. You've got the will and spirit to overcome this. There's no question that you'll get better with time."

I hugged her and told her that she was really good at this "for better or for worse" thing, and that it was she who kept my spirits up.

"I'll tell you what," I said. When I get better and can walk on my own again, I'll take you to the Caribbean or somewhere where there is a wide sandy beach and the water is bright turquoise and the mojitos flow endlessly from marble fountains and we'll celebrate together."

"That's a deal."

By the time Terri said good night, I felt better, and resolved to focus my attention on physical therapy until my nerves started to regenerate.

Just as FDR's "Day that will Live in Infamy" speech is embedded in the national conscience, Howard's "marathon, not a sprint" speech became part of our mantra while I was on the mend.

10 A Plateau on Two Mountains

A few days before my release from the hospital, a team of physical and occupational therapists (consisting of Beth, Sarah, and Michelle) took me back to my apartment to determine any necessary modifications that I would need to get around. Terri came too.

I hadn't gotten any weaker in my month at the hospital, but I wasn't gaining strength either. I seemed a ghostly image of my former self. My arms and legs looked emaciated. If I tried to wave to anyone my wrists drooped, an embarrassment. So I didn't wave. I couldn't clap my hands because my finger muscles didn't work, so I avoided clapping. I needed special key chains to use a door key. On my feet, I wore plastic ankle flexion orthotics, called AFO's, to counteract my foot drop. These fit into my shoes and rose up midway between my ankles and knees. A plain white velcro strap kept them tight around my legs. Pretty unsightly when I wore shorts, but in warm weather I wore them anyway, burying my vanity. Search as we did, Terri and I were unable to find more stylish orthotics. I'm certain there is a fortune to be made in designing snazzy, colorful AFOs.

Luckily, our apartment building on upper Connecticut Avenue was well suited for wheelchair use. The wheelchair entrance was on a side street just off Connecticut Avenue. A ramp led to the door that gave access to a hallway on the second floor. I could gain entry by swiping the lock with my magnetic key and then pushing the handicap button for the door to open. I had to back the chair up to allow room for the door to swing open, but once I had my motorized chair I'd get used to that.

When we arrived at the apartment, Beth asked me to try to walk down the ramp to the side door rather than her wheeling me in the chair. At that time, the motorized chair was on order, so we were using a regular wheelchair. The idea was for me to walk with my rolling walker to the ramp and then place my hands on the iron rails on either side of the ramp. The ramp was not steep, but the rails were too low for me to take hold of without bending my knees. I made a game effort, but my legs were much too weak for me to bend even slightly, so I called for the chair. I started to perspire from the stress of my failed effort while, at the same time, I felt humiliated that I couldn't manage such a simple feat. Beth tried to console me with the thought that I was likely tired from the trip home that had involved a lesson in transferring in and out of the passenger seat of the car from my wheel chair. I knew better.

Our eighth floor apartment had two bedrooms with a narrow hall leading from the living room back to the bedrooms. It was clear that I would need to use my walker in tandem with the chair. The thick carpeting made it difficult for me to wheel myself in the manual chair, but I anticipated the arrival of my motorized chair within a few weeks. I could guide a motorized chair slowly through the hallways into my bedroom, but the entrances to either bathroom were too narrow for any type of chair. There would be no option but for me to walk to the bathroom. Same with the narrow galley kitchen.

Once in the apartment, Beth and Michelle made some instant pronouncements while Sarah took notes. Since I would be working part time from home while Terri went to her office, I would need to be self-sufficient. Terri would have to take up the throw rugs that complimented our wall-to-wall carpeting. These would only serve to trip me when I needed to use my walker to enter the kitchen or bathrooms. We would purchase a mechanical lift chair to allow me to stand and grab hold of the walker. By simply pressing a button, the lift chair would rise up and tilt forward, allowing me to pop up and reach for my walker. The sofa and other chairs were off limit as someone would have to lift me out of them. Beth planned to give Terri a lesson on how to lift me without destroying her back on my last day before being released from the hospital.

Anticipating my homecoming, we'd attached a small basket to my walker, much like the baskets used to attach to the handlebars of a bike, so that I could keep with me essentials like a phone and other stuff I needed. Michelle examined the fridge and kitchen cabinets. Terri was to make sure before she left for the day that my lunch and other food items I needed would be within easy reach. Juice or milk would be in plastic glasses or cups that I could handle. It took both of my hands to grip a glass so there was no way that I could hold the door to the fridge open and lift a carton of juice or milk. I never did master the skill necessary to use the long grabber that the therapists had tried to get me to use to reach stuff that was high up. Therefore, items I knew I would need, such as coffee, had to be handy. The plan was for me to take my walker into the kitchen, put it to the side, lean against the side of the fridge for balance, reach for my lunch or drink, place either on the counter, and walk around the counter to the chairs facing it. Fortunately, we owned tall counter chairs that I could get in and out of on my own. My routine would be to rise from my lift chair into my walker, shuffle to the kitchen or bathroom, and then back to the lift chair. I couldn't have imagined such a life a mere three months before.

For Terri, every morning before she'd leave for work would be like preparing for a space launch, checking that no detail was overlooked: my juice poured and placed in the fridge so that I'd be able to reach it and my lunch made and left on the counter. Everything I'd need throughout the day in easy reach. Nothing could be left in my way. In truth, Terri was as anxious about my return home as she had been at her first court hearing, although she didn't express it. I'd been well cared for at the hospital by doctors, nurses, and countless tech aides. Now, my wellbeing depended solely on Terri who had a very full and stressful day job. It wasn't going to be a waltz through the park. And we both knew it.

With the home visit completed, Sarah wheeled me back to Beth's car for the drive back to the hospital. Terri headed to the metro to go back to work. It was a gorgeous, bright spring day and I longed to be out and about on my own steam. On the way to the car, we ran into a neighbor of ours, a retired, older woman named Charlotte. She looked puzzled. My downhill spiral before I entered the hospital had occurred so rapidly that not all of my acquaintances knew of my condition. I felt the same need to explain my distressed circumstance as I would have if I were being led away in an orange jumpsuit with handcuffs and shackles.

"Hi Charlotte, I've been in the hospital for several weeks. Did you know?"

"No, no, I had no idea," she said, without disguising her astonishment. "I knew you were having some difficulty with balance, but you were walking."

"Yes, but my neuropathy—no one knows the cause, but it got worse. I expect to get better, though. I'll be home in a couple of days." An awkward exchange. I nodded to Beth and we headed back to her car.

We drove in silence through neighborhoods where I'd taken so many strolls before. Down Connecticut Avenue through the bustling commercial strip of Cleveland Park, past the National Zoo, across the bridge over Rock Creek Park. Tulips bloomed on the small park square at the intersection of Connecticut and Kalorama. We turned off Connecticut, just north of Dupont Circle, back toward the hospital.

During my last couple of days in rehab, therapy focused on practical concerns surrounding my ability to function on my own at home. Toward that end, Sarah attempted to teach me how to get myself off the floor in case I fell. At her urging, I pushed myself backward on my butt toward an exercise bed that stood about three feet high. So far, so good. Then, she instructed me to get on my knees and turn facing the bed. I did that. "Now, place both arms on the bed and pull yourself up onto it in stages, first one knee up, then the other," she said.

Try as I would, I just didn't have the strength to pull myself up.

I tried pulling myself up on my stomach. That didn't work either. "I guess I better not fall," I said.

Next, she had me walk in my walker and push aside any obstacles that lay in my path. She placed several items, large and small, in my way. I fared a little better at this task. I pushed aside one large item with my right hand. Then, returning my hand to the walker, I took another step. And so on. I shoved small items strewn around the floor out of the way with my foot. Not easy, but I could do it.

Michelle had me practice in the rehab unit's makeshift kitchen, opening and removing items from the fridge or taking items from cabinet shelves. I had to learn to be careful and patient. No shortcuts or I'd stumble and fall. Then we went outdoors with my wheelchair. I donned bicycle gloves to make it easier to grip the wheels. I strained to wheel myself up the ramp and down the street along the sidewalk. I managed to roll a half block, but so slowly and strenuously that it hardly seemed worth the effort.

In truth, I too was nervous about returning home, especially since I wasn't getting better. If Terri was at work, I couldn't call for a nurse's aide should I get into trouble. Each morning when I woke in the hospital I'd cautiously study my condition. I don't seem to be worse, I'd tell myself. Nor any better. I guess that I've reached what the doctors called a plateau. I comforted myself with the notion that this was like Kilimanjaro where we spent several days circling the mountain at 12-13,000 feet before attempting the final ascent to the summit.

We had arrived at Barranco Camp, at 13,000 feet, on the late afternoon of the third day of our climb. We'd been descending for the previous hour, and found ourselves in the upper reaches of the Alpine Moorland climate zone, a region of grasslands, rocks, gravel, beautiful flowers, and stunted shrubbery. Senecio plants dotted the landscape. Sometimes referred to as Groundsels (a more descriptive term), these plants are rounded with pale green flat leaves jutting out on all sides like sharp spikes. Mostly, they grow from the ground, but occasionally they emerge in clusters from the heads of what appear to be rubber stalks, perhaps eight feet or more in height. Looking at these bizarre plants, it is easy to imagine one has been transported to another planet.

As we entered the camp area, directly ahead of us, on the far side of the camp, loomed an imposing and intimidating sight—the Great Barranco Breach Wall. This immense granite rock stretched as wide and far as I could see, posing a formidable obstacle to proceeding onward with the climb. It was unmistakable that to go beyond our camp, in the direction in which we had been walking, we would have to negotiate this wall.

"How do we get around it?" I wondered out loud, knowing full well the answer.

"We don't," Ray and Lisa said in unison. "We go up and over it first thing in the morning."

We were now in a segment of the climb during which we would be maintaining pretty much the same altitude for several days—a plateau. It would take another three plus days, and three more camps, before we would make the final nighttime ascent.

On the previous day, having left the rain forest behind, we'd traversed paths of dirt and scree (small pebbles) amidst giant heather, tall trees, and lovely flowering plants, such as the native pink Protea, with pointy leaves circling its fuzzy center. We had scrambled up jagged rocks for about two hours. Terri and I were thankful that we had practiced a rock scramble the previous autumn at a popular destination known as Old Rag, in the Shenandoah Valley of western Virginia. When this time we pulled ourselves up the very last rock, we emerged at the Shira Plateau, a vast open expanse at the higher edge of the Alpine Moorland Zone.

At this elevation tall trees and heather gradually give way to gravel, rocks, and boulders. Vegetation is thinner, the plant life being reduced to lichen and scattered tufts of grass peeking out between the rocks. The air here, on this second day of the climb, was crisp and cool under a bright cloudless sky. Although I was perspiring a little from the rock scramble, I was exhilarated, enjoying myself far more than I had the previous day when I had been clumsily groping my way uphill through the rain forest.

It was on the Shira Plateau, for the first time since we'd begun our trek, when the majestic volcanic summit of Kilimanjaro came into full view. Hemingway's description of the mountain in his short story *The Snows of Kilimanjaro*, came to mind. "...there, ahead, as wide as all the world, great, high, and unbelievably white in the sun, was the top of Kilimanjaro." Our view, undoubtedly, took in less "white" than Hemingway had beheld. The summit appeared vast, to be sure, an immense wall of rock dissected by slivers of white glaciers, but perhaps not quite so "unbelievably white." Photos taken over the past century, indeed, confirm that the snows of Kilimanjaro have been receding.

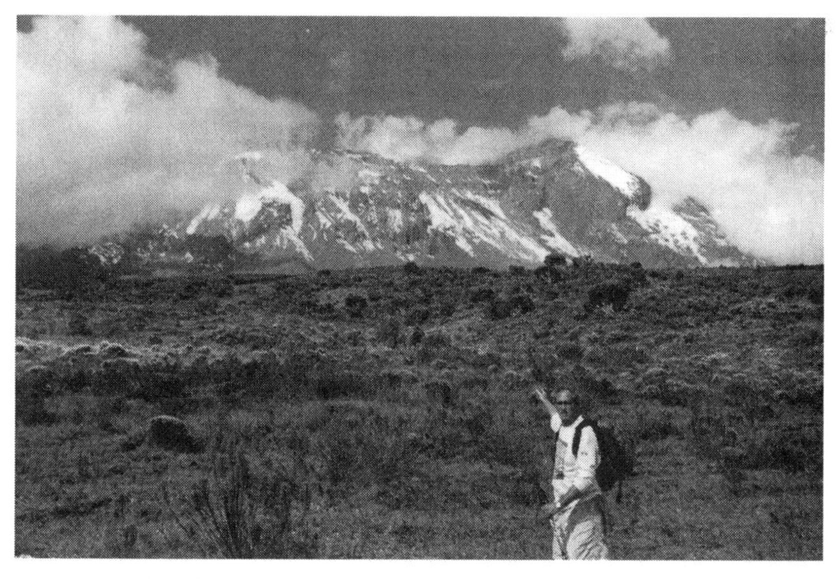

Michael below Kilimanjaro's snow-capped summit
two days before the all night ascent

The plan called for us to camp the second night a little higher up on the Shira Plateau, at 12,500 feet. Then, for the following two days, we would circle the summit, perhaps one fifth of the way around, camping at around 13,000 feet both nights. Plateauing (not gaining altitude) for these next few days would help us acclimate to the higher altitude, so we wouldn't get sick and die, say, of a cerebral edema.

On the final day of our upward push we would ascend to 15,500 feet where we'd make camp. Then we'd be permitted but a few hours nap time before beginning our assault on the summit that same night. After reaching the top (assuming success, of course, for we could not allow ourselves to think otherwise), we'd be allowed to savor the scene for about a half hour before beginning the long trek back down the mountain.

As we set out for Shira Camp, Ray noticed that the top of my forehead had turned bright red. "Michael, didn't you bring a hat; this equatorial sun will roast you."

"Yes, but it's in my duffle, I'm afraid. Yesterday there was no sun at all, so I didn't give it much thought."

"Oh Michael," Terri said, "you have to protect your head." I knew full well that a hat or visor was on the list of required items to bring.

Lisa came to the rescue. "I have a bandana in my pack. Here, wear this," she said as she pulled out a red and white scarf.

Terri tied the bandana around my head as we forged ahead toward camp. "Now, with your headdress and hair stubble, you truly look like a rugged mountain man," she said, as we proceeded toward camp.

At Shira Camp, nearby slopes and hills partially hid the mountaintop from view. Dusk altered the array of colors of the landscape around us. The gray and white of the rock and snow that had marked the summit earlier had become less sharply defined, the gray now melded to a golden brown and the white of the glaciers faded to a silvery gray. The nearby slopes also took on a golden hue with the plant growth a markedly darker green or yellow in the moonlight.

At some point over 13,000 feet, the landscape shifts from Alpine moorland to Alpine desert. As we started our upward climb the third morning of our adventure, instead of stunted plant growth, we soon found ourselves traversing a region of rocks and boulders and loose scree, absent of vegetation. It was like wandering on the moon or another distant world; we saw only desert and rocks in every direction. We kept a steady pace, stopping for water breaks now and then. The landscape shifted back and forth between desert and moorland as we ascended and dipped over the terrain, skirting rocks and boulders. There were no rock scrambles or other great challenges this day, just a long steady push forward, up and down, toward Barranco Camp. The loose scree could be slippery in those parts where the undulating trail wound downward. On several occasions I made a deliberate choice to slide downhill on my butt rather than risk a tumble.

A long, albeit not steep, descent toward Barranco Camp brought us back into a region of Alpine moorland with plants and shrubbery again in abundance. And, ahead, in the distance, instilling in me a sense of foreboding, loomed the Great Barranco Breach Wall.

The next morning (our third day) we headed straight for the wall. We were relieved to see people, looking like tiny specks in the distance, scaling it in single file. Perhaps our task would not be so treacherous after all. In about two hours we reached the wall. Steps had been carved into the rocks making the first part of our ascent easy enough. James led the way and the rest of us kept single file behind him. The porters, lugging all of our gear, had long since passed us. Before long, the steps became fewer and farther between, and the climb turned into another rock scramble. Every so often I'd look up at what seemed to be the very top of the wall and my spirits would lift. These visions invariably turned out to be false. Several times I reached what I thought was the last stretch, only to see more granite rising high above. As with Sisyphus, the mythical character who'd hauled heavy rocks for eternity, it seemed our ordeal would never end.

"*Polé, polé,*" I recalled the porters' refrain. Take it slowly. One step, then another. And then we came to this ledge, a moment I shan't forget:

The ledge is so narrow that we must hug the rock in front of us while shuffling along sideways. I place my hands on the wall and rest my chin against it. Then slowly and gingerly I move my feet to the place where James is waiting. I'm acutely aware that if I turn to look behind me, I'd see a precipitous drop of several hundred feet. Still, I can't help but take a peek. Quickly, I turn back to again face the wall, tightening my grip. Never mind the scrapes. I'm not ready to die.

"Don't look down, whatever you do," Lisa and Terri warned.

"I already did," I said.

"Figures."

James is waiting at a small crevice, and as we reach him, one by one, he helps us across. Steep steps ahead tell us we still have a ways to go. We pull ourselves up these rocks, and after what seems an eternity we reach the top of the wall.

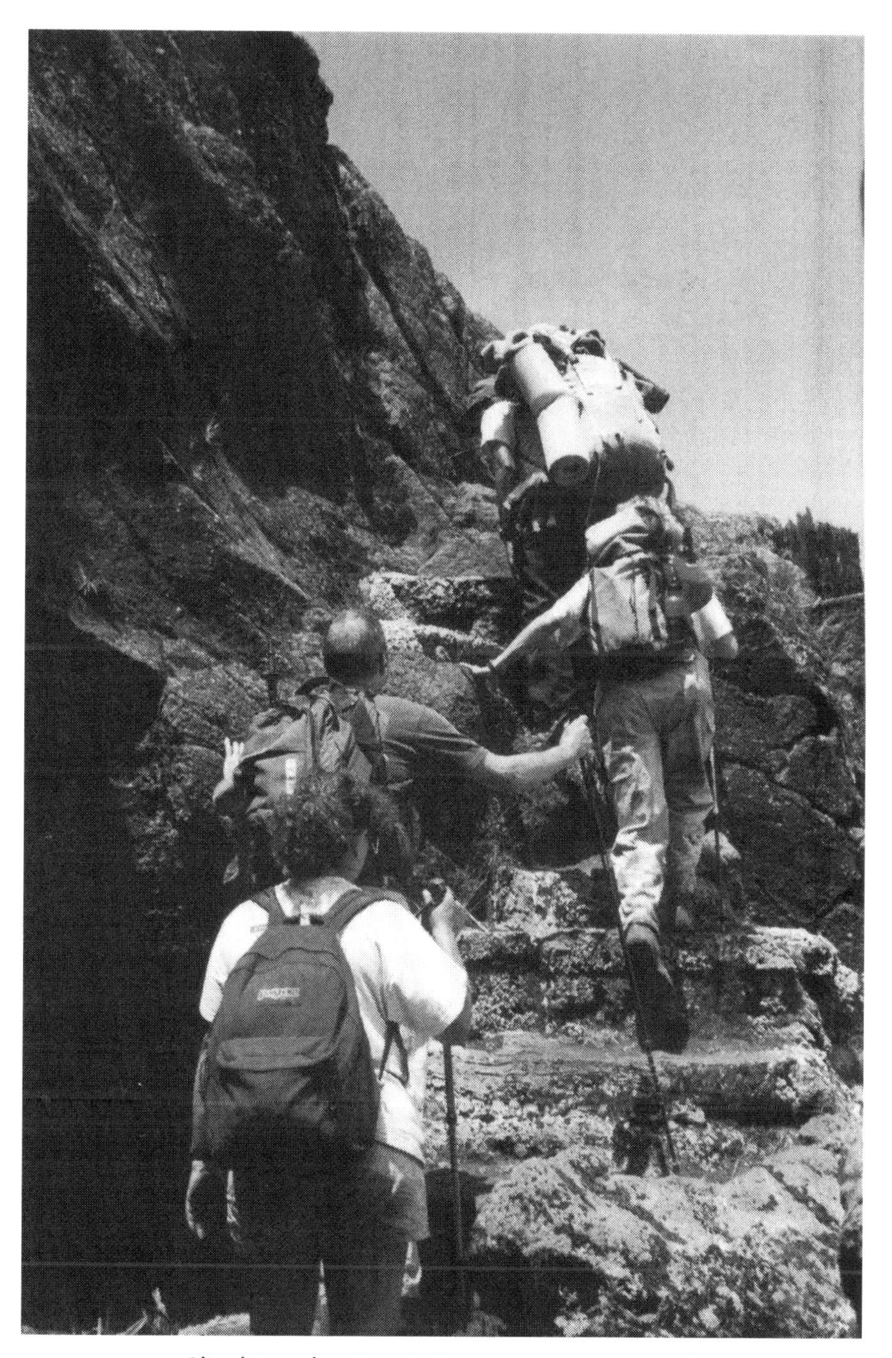

Climbing the Great Barranco Breach Wall

"That was like three or four Old Rags rolled into one," I said to anyone who'd listen.

"Old Rag was a playpen compared to this," Terri said. I recalled that many of the day-trippers who had huffed and puffed up Old Rag had seemed woefully out of shape.

After resting, we continued along a trail on relatively flat ground, arriving at Karanga camp by mid-afternoon. For the third straight night, we made camp at about 13,000 feet. We found ourselves the only group stopping at this place, most others having forged ahead to the last camp, Barafu Camp, at 15,500 feet. We had not gained altitude over the past two days, but, hopefully, this meant we'd be less inclined toward altitude sickness as we prepared to make the final ascent.

Karanga Camp was set in a region of moorland with a variety of plant growth including clusters of grass, shrubs, and yellow flowers evident all around. Stunted tree trunks stood in some places, drooping like old folks whose bones had curved with age. This was a landscape stressed by centuries of wind and cold.

Leaving Lisa and Ray to rest, or write cards in their tent, Terri and I took a stroll after teatime. We walked along a stream where the porters were cooling a supply of bottled water. The summit was partially in view, a little closer to us now than on previous nights. The setting sun gave dramatic effect to the shades of charcoal of the mountain, the faded white of the glaciers, the dark shadows of the volcanic rocks, and the surrounding landscape of green and golden slopes dotted with wild flowers and shrubs. We gazed in wonder at the mountaintop which at long last we would tackle the following night. It was difficult to know how we would fare on the final ascent. It would be a tough go, but this was what we'd been looking forward to and toiling toward over the past few days; indeed, the past several months. We felt a degree of excitement and a degree of trepidation.

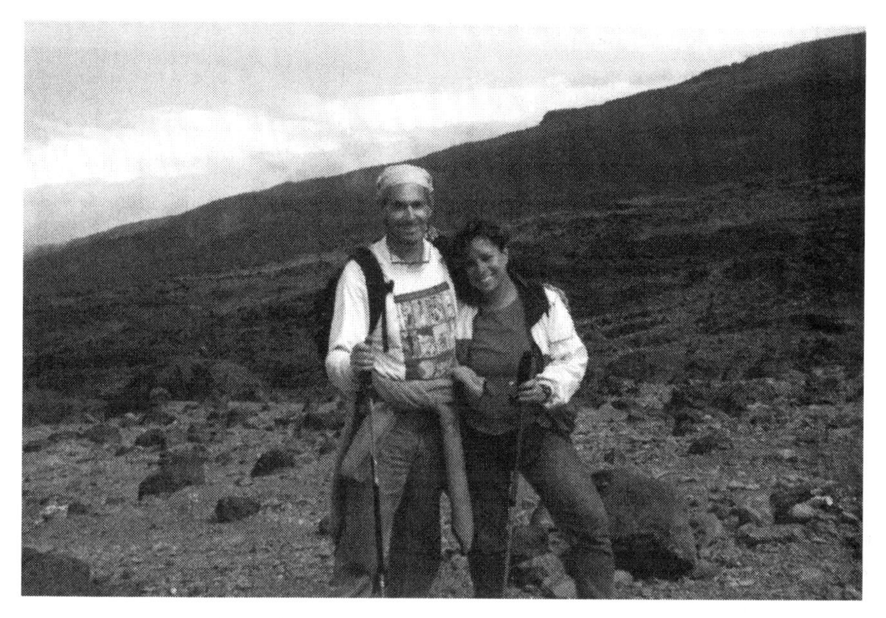

Terri and Michael on the upper slopes of Kilimanjaro

Heading back to our tent, we paused to take photos of the porters who were laughing and telling stories in Swahili while preparing dinner over a fire. They happily posed for the camera.

"I've been bothered by a slight headache," Terri confided to me as we stooped to enter our tent.

"Take some Diamox now, and we'll see how you feel in the morning." Diamox was the medicine prescribed for minor symptoms of altitude sickness, such as headaches. However, if such symptoms persisted or got worse, there was no option but to descend.

"I'd hate to quit now," Terri said. "We've been doing so well."

"Take the Diamox and the chances are you'll be fine tomorrow."

As we lay down in our sleeping bags we could faintly hear the porters singing tribal songs and conversing, their words punctuated by occasional bursts of laughter. Exhaustion led to sleep. We knew we would not sleep the next night, or, perhaps, not until we got back to Arusha.

Back home in my new reality, I suddenly understood plateau metaphors in a whole different way. Once I got home from the hospital for good, I settled into a daily routine that entailed my working four hours a day, a compromise I'd worked out with my office. I reviewed documents, typed notes on the computer, and composed motions and memoranda. Although I kept in touch with my office by phone and email, I missed the personal interaction with the folks there. I also didn't want to use up too much more of my accumulated sick leave. I resolved to return to the office as soon as I got my motorized chair.

I tried to be careful getting around the apartment, but I did suffer one mishap during my first week home. One morning, after Terri had left for work, I tumbled on my way out of the bathroom. I was okay, but the walker turned over and the mobile phone fell out of the basket. After uttering a dozen or so curses, I somehow managed to pull myself backward and up onto the toilet commode. Sarah would have been proud. I then reached for the walker and righted it, but the phone was beyond my reach. Using the handrails on the commode, I rose into the walker and made my way to the wall phone in the kitchen. I phoned Charlotte who lived in the neighboring apartment and whom I thought might be home. She came over and retrieved the phone, but she expressed concern about my having to rely on her for assistance. Another reason why I looked forward to going back to the office: It would be safer than staying home alone.

Eighteen months. I'd better start getting better soon.

11 Billie

One of my marching orders while Terri was at work was to try my damnedest not to tumble again. She'd arranged things in the apartment much as we'd planned when Beth and Sarah had made their home visit several weeks before. She'd removed the throw rugs and placed our new mechanical lift chair by a wall outlet opposite the sofa, partially facing the TV. I wasn't a fan of daytime TV anyway. The walker would always be at my side, mobile phone in the basket, so I could rise from the chair, step into the walker, and safely get to my computer in the bedroom, or the kitchen to make coffee, or fetch my ready-made lunch. My wheelchair was also accessible although the weakness of my finger and wrist muscles made it difficult to maneuver on the carpet.

As I think back, I can recall how frustrating it was to come home and strategize my every move. On one level I knew I was in a marathon, but in my gut I wanted to sprint to the finish. Being impatient wasn't helping me cope. On Kilimanjaro it was the soccer players, the athletic types who scrambled up the mountain as fast as they could—it was they who had the greatest difficulty reaching the summit. The altitude was their undoing. Patience and perseverance had been our reward then. I'd do well to remember that now.

One day during my first week home, I was sitting at the kitchen counter drinking my third cup of coffee of the morning, both of my hands cradling the mug, when the phone rang. I lifted the phone from the basket attached to the walker. The woman's voice on the other end was very soft.

"Hello, is this Samuel?" Apparently, my hospital records, like other official documents, used my full name from my birth certificate.

" I go by Michael," I said. "Who is this?"

"This is Billie. I'd like to schedule your physical therapy. I have your papers from the discharge nurse." I could detect a slight accent that I couldn't decipher.

Between her accent and the faintness of her voice, I had to strain to understand her.

" I just got out of the hospital," I said. "Can we do this next week, perhaps?" I didn't want to deal with much of anything just yet. Feeling my way back into my new daily routine without the full use of my arms and legs was enough to handle. While the hospital discharge instructions called for intensive and frequent therapy sessions, everything was too much at once. Figuring out how to cope on my own in our two-bedroom condo apartment while my wife went to work was sufficiently daunting. Working therapy sessions into my life would have to wait. Just leave me alone, I wanted to shout, but didn't. What still escaped me was that without hard work through therapy, any recovery, if it were to happen, would take longer.

"We can start next week if you prefer, but let's set it up now," Billie said.

"I can't go anywhere on my own now. And my wife works all day."

"I can come to your house in the evenings. Would Tuesdays and Thursdays work for you?"

I was running out of excuses. "Okay," I grumbled. "About seven?"

"Yes, I'll come next Tuesday at seven."

"But just physical therapy," I said. "Not occupational therapy."

"No, someone will call to schedule occupational therapy separately." She mentioned a name but I never got that call, which suited me fine.

The following Tuesday, Billie came as arranged. In light of her soft-spoken voice on the phone, I was surprised by her appearance. She was a tall, dark-skinned Ugandan woman about 40 years old, I guessed. She was the kind of woman you'd notice when she walked into a room, regal with an amazing wardrobe of glittery shirts and spiked heels. She kept her eyebrows pencil-thin and well arched, and had shiny gloss on her wide lips. She still had family in Uganda as well as all over the United States and the rest of the world. We later learned that in Uganda, Billie was an actual princess. "I almost went to medical school," she told us. "But in the end, I liked to party too much." I was dazzled by her painted and matching finger and toenails: bright turquoise with gold and black squiggles, or pink with blue markings. She seemed to change the colors and design every time she came.

On this first visit, she wanted to discuss the nature of my illness and then test my muscles and determine my level of functioning.

"What exactly is your condition?" she asked.

"My diagnosis is CIDP," I explained, for what seemed the millionth time. In the hospital it seemed every medical intern or resident pressed me for an explanation of my illness. The doctors explained my condition to each new group of medical students accompanying them on their rounds. So I knew the drill. But while the doctors had been optimistic that in time my nerves would regenerate, albeit slowly, the therapists who did their homework and read about my diagnosis tended to be more skeptical. They'd stress the uncertainty of my outcome and that I'd need to work my muscles every day. I hated that; I longed for assurance that I'd get back to normal without all that extra effort. For Billie's benefit, I launched into my own assessment of my condition.

"The experimental treatments didn't seem to be working for me," I told her. "So, I've suffered serious damage to my peripheral nerves. As a result, I can't get up on my own from a sitting position, nor can I effectively use my hands." I went on to tell her that for now I was quadriplegic, but that the prognosis for some level of recovery was generally good because the nerves regenerate and potentially may reconnect with the muscles.

Echoing Terri's Uncle Howard, I explained that the extent of recovery varies greatly among patients and that the question of what treatments would work was uncertain.

"If you are willing to work hard at physical therapy the odds for getting better will increase in your favor." I'd heard that before, but perhaps I needed to hear it again and again.

Billie didn't work me too hard on that first visit and kept it short. Maybe this wouldn't be so bad after all.

She came again that Thursday evening. "What caused the CIDP? " she asked. It was clear she'd done some reading about my illness over the past two days.

"The docs don't really know," I said. "It's considered idiopathic. In fact, my diagnosis is called 'Idiopathic CIDP.'" Then I told her that it might have something do with Africa since we'd been there just four months before I started experiencing symptoms. I recalled that none of the neurologists thought that our trip to Africa had any connection to my illness; they considered four months too much of a time lapse to suspect any of the inoculations I had gotten for the trip. However, Dr. Sherman had had a different view. He had told me that his hunch—and he had emphasized that it was only a hunch—was that my CIDP was somehow linked to our trip, possibly the high altitude in climbing Kilimanjaro.

"In truth, nobody has a clue. But I'm supposed to get better," I insisted.

"As I said the other day, one way to get better while your nerves are trying to regenerate is through physical therapy. We will start with the straight leg raises." Billie took it easy with me the first couple of visits gently testing the parameters of my strength and endurance. Terri would be there too if she didn't have to work late. During our third or fourth session, in order to test my balance, Billie had me stand up in my walker for 10 seconds without holding on. I recall that moment quite well:

I crank the lift chair all the way up and forward so that it is practically spitting me out like a dead clam. I stand up straight, placing first my left and then my right hand on each side of the metal frame of the walker and step into it. Billie tells me to let go of the walker, one hand at a time and then both hands at the same time. When I place both hands by my side she starts to count. One, two.... That's as far as I get. My knees are slightly bent and I feel myself about to drop to the floor so I again grip the walker with both hands and straighten my posture. We repeat this exercise several times, but I don't manage to get beyond the count of four. My foot balance is virtually nonexistent. "We will try again next time," Billie says. If only I had her patience.

I was reminded of our first day on the Kilimanjaro climb, in the rain forest, when I'd had a dismal time keeping my footing on the slick muddy ground.

"What's the matter?" our guide, James, had asked.

"It's just slippery," I'd said. After we completed the climb and were celebrating our success over beers with the porters, James confided that he never thought our little group of four would reach the summit. He saved his supreme compliment for me.

"That first day, Michael, you were walking like drunk man."

"And you thought that was water in my flask," I shot back. We all laughed, including the porters, after James interpreted our remarks for them. We'd all been a little clumsy from time to time, and were constantly in awe of the ability of the porters to make it all seem so simple. There we'd been, each of us adventurers, with a day pack and ski pole, in our mud-caked hiking boots, climbing and stumbling our way up the mountain, while the porters had passed right by us balancing our tents, luggage, and food on their heads, dressed in K-mart quality shorts and sandals or flip flops, and not carrying any kind of walking stick.

"*Jambo*," they'd say good-naturedly, as they sauntered by.

"*Jambo*," we'd answer back, and then laugh and scowl about how easy it all seemed for them when they were out of earshot.

As my second week of home therapy sessions ended, I wished I had just a little of the balance that I had had during that first day of the climb in the rain forest.

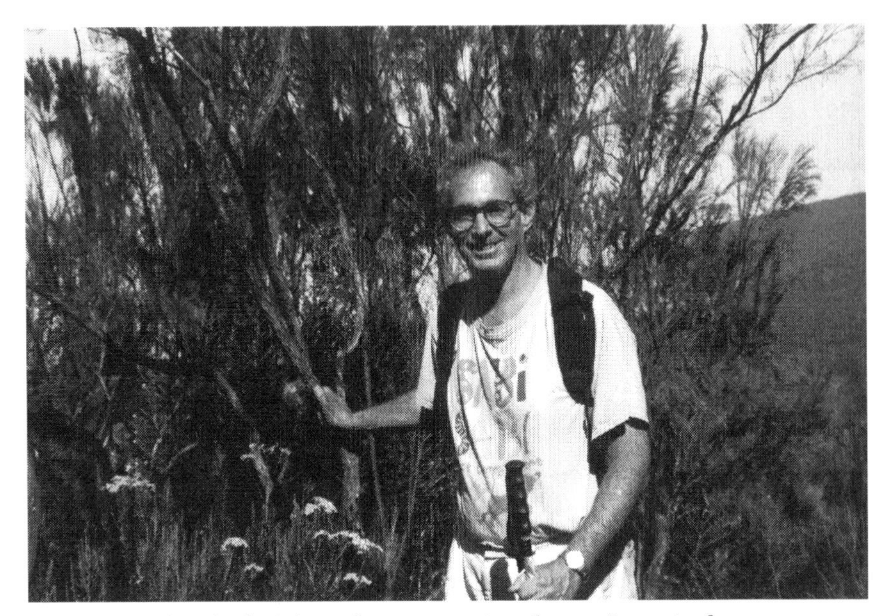

Michael, the day after emerging from the rain forest

There were times when I couldn't understand Billie she spoke so quietly. "Today, we will walk fast," she said to me one day during my third or fourth week of sessions. Billie usually wanted to test my walking before I got tired from the other exercises.

"But Billie, I can't walk fast." Terri laughed at my confusion.

"We will walk FIRST," Billie repeated, dragging out the "r" sound in her Ugandan accent.

"Oh, FIRST. I see. Okay then, let's get the walking out of the way." Another time, Billie took me into the bedroom for exercises. She had prescribed a regimen of strength exercises involving use of leg weights and dumbbells that I did lying face up or sitting on the bed. This time, after I completed my routine, she asked me to stay on the bed and try different maneuvers: roll over, sit up, balance on my knees, like a puppy learning new tricks. Although it wasn't Billie's intent—at least we didn't think so at the time—Terri and I considered these exercises a precursor to the re-emergence of sex in our lives. Prior to my illness we had enjoyed a vibrant life in the sack, but there is nothing like a bout with quadriplegia to stifle both the interest and ability to perform.

Billie's intent was to train my muscles to be ready to perform as they had in the past when, and if, I regained sufficient strength. "Make your muscles ready to work for you," she would often say.

"Let's see if you can rise up on all fours like a dog." I could do that.

"Now, try to get all the way up."

"Are you kidding?"

"Even if you can't get all the way up now, the muscles need to get used to your making the effort. Don't try this on your own, but we will practice again next session."

Billie showed great patience and a mature sense of how to challenge me. Despite her quiet demeanor, she was no softy and always found new challenges by utilizing the resources at her disposal. She didn't need all the gadgets and equipment they had at the hospital. She made innovative use of whatever objects she found in our apartment building, like the stairs in the lobby. Also, I trusted her more than the young therapists at GW who often just followed the regimen given to them. Except for Beth. I'd liked and trusted Beth very much because she would challenge me at every opportunity. I looked forward to the day when I could walk again, and would go back to the PT unit at the hospital and find Beth and show her how well I had done. I didn't know how long that would be, but I was certain that I would walk again. I told Billie that often in my dreams I'd start to walk or even jog. "Seeing yourself walk in your dreams is a good sign," she said more than once.

After several sessions, I mustered the courage to ask Billie whether *she* thought that I would ever walk again. She was unequivocal: "You have shown that you are willing to work hard and you walk with Terri every day, so I have confidence that you will be walking before long."

She then told me about a client of hers, a robust lady who had a condition similar to mine, but who was content to live life in her motorized wheelchair. "Try as I did, she refused to walk. She mostly watched TV and relied on her family for everything. I couldn't convince her to take therapy seriously. As far as I know, she never improved. She didn't care. But you aren't like her. You will get better. When the weather is good, we will go outside and walk around the block."

"Go outdoors, I like that idea," Terri chimed in.

"I do too," I said, but inwardly I felt terrified.

Billie knew I'd be going back to the office as soon as my motorized chair arrived. The plan was for Terri, who worked in the same building, to drive me to and from work, leaving in time for evening therapy sessions. I explained that while I'd be fine going to work downtown, what I'd miss would be the travel that is a big part of my casework. "That would be too difficult until I could walk and function independently," I said. "So I'll have to delegate my travel to a colleague."

"What do your cases involve?" Billie asked.

I explained as best I could, telling her about my early days in civil rights to my current work on environmental tort cases. Billie was actually quite interested in what I had to say. "Civil Rights," I explained, "involved prosecuting cases, whereas now I defend the government when aggrieved people sue because of personal injury or property damage."

When I began working in the Torts Branch in 1984, the office was consumed by the asbestos litigation. Because we were able to rebuff the efforts of the asbestos companies to make the government partially responsibility for the harm caused by their products, the mission of the office gradually shifted to defending toxic tort cases. I proceeded to tell Billie about one such case I worked on for a full decade beginning in the late 80's.

The case was brought by more than 60 families in Jacksonville, Florida, who claimed that chemical waste from two naval air stations had been dumped at a private landfill in their neighborhood, causing a myriad of symptoms and illnesses. The scenario brings to mind such motion pictures as *A Civil Action* and *Erin Brokovich*. Here, however, I was convinced that the injury claims were greatly inflated, if not altogether bogus. Any community suffers from a variety of illnesses; there appeared to be nothing out of the ordinary among those Jacksonville residents.

Partly because of my achievements working on the asbestos litigation, the office asked me to assume the role of lead counsel on the Jacksonville case. I accepted the role but had little idea what I was getting into. The case, which took ten years to resolve, had many twists and turns, involved several trials and evidentiary hearings, testimony by scores of fact witnesses, and testimony by experts in such varied fields as toxicology, epidemiology, groundwater hydrology, and several medical specialties. The case also involved give and take with a feisty and at times cranky federal judge, and the efforts over a full decade of dozens of lawyers in my office, some with large egos, working under my direction. Being lead counsel on a case this size was a little like directing a movie with a cast of prima donna actors. The task required the juggling of competing interests, schedules, and a variety of other complex factors.

The first big trial took place in early 1992 and lasted nine weeks, eight in the sterile federal courthouse in downtown Jacksonville and the final week in an elegant old county courthouse in Daytona Beach. It was biker week at Daytona, and I found it difficult to get much sleep with the continuous roar of the cycles revving up all through the night. At the end of the trial the judge found the government at fault, but awarded minimum damages because he held that most of the injury claims had nothing to do with the landfill. There would be more issues to resolve, however, and more trials and hearings before the case would end. I was a boxer going 15 rounds, staggering to my corner after round three.

The trial came at a busy time. During this period, Jessica was living with me, her mom having died two years earlier. While I was away at trial, she stayed with teachers during the school week and with good friends on the weekends. I distributed a lengthy memo detailing all the essential information: phone numbers, addresses, the names of those who would transport her from one place to another, etc. I also needed to get her into a less restrictive school because of the progress she'd made. And I needed to move my mother from Miami to a nursing home near me. I was juggling.

When I say that the judge in the case could be feisty and cranky, this may be an understatement. One time, I sent a young lawyer to Jacksonville to conduct a short evidentiary hearing. I believed he was ready for this assignment. During the hearing the judge was having difficulty finding documents in the evidence notebook that plaintiffs' lawyers had provided. At one point, our lawyer approached the podium to address the court. The judge proceeded to holler at him for a full ten minutes because of his frustration with the other side's notebook. I guess you might say that our young lawyer received his baptism by fire that day.

The judge took a particular delight in excoriating expert witnesses who he believed were less than objective in their opinions. "Hired guns" was his term for such witnesses. He blamed both sides for sponsoring hired guns, often with ample justification. One time a medical expert for the plaintiffs testified about the cost of certain medical monitoring procedures that plaintiffs sought to be awarded due to what they claimed was an increased risk of cancer. On cross-examination it turned out that the doctor had relied on information provided by the plaintiffs' law firm to support his testimony. The judge, furious at this revelation, turned to the expert and said something like: "You might be an esteemed member of the medical profession doctor, but if you would rely on information supplied by a paralegal, you are also a member of what is commonly referred to as the world's oldest profession." That was the last we heard from that expert.

After ten years, when we could at long last celebrate victory, I quipped that I might sue the office for causing my hair to turn from brown to gray as a result of this case. Never mind that my hair color might have been impacted by the fact that I was forty when the case was filed and fifty when in 1997 I finally managed to get the trial court decisions that had gone against us reversed by a federal appeals court in Atlanta. In the end, I suppose that one lesson I took from this experience was the reward gained from perseverance.

"Perseverance," Billie repeated, as I concluded my story. "That's a good lesson for you in dealing with your illness."

Billie was intensely interested in American politics and had educated herself on recent American history. She detested Republicans. "I can't understand why Americans elected an actor and a not very good one at that," she said one day as she tightened the Velcro straps on my leg weights.

"Once upon a time I was a Republican," I said.

"No way," she grimaced.

I explained that except for Uncle Lou, a political agnostic, my New York family was totally Republican. I recalled walking up Broadway as a little tike, my mother in tow, proudly displaying the "I like Ike" button pinned on my t-shirt. When we got to the polling place, the lady in charge opened the curtain to the voting booth and allowed me to go inside with my mother. I pulled the lever for Ike and Nixon. I also remember my cousin Patsy dancing around the dining room table singing a little ditty: "Whistle while you work, Nixon is a jerk, Eisenhower's got the power, Stevenson is turning sour, whistle while you work."

"But you were very young, you didn't know better." Billie laughed.

"Maybe, but I also remember rooting for Nixon against Kennedy when I was 13. I kept hoping Nixon would pull it out when, in the aftermath of the election, votes were re-counted in Ohio and Texas. Even in high school I sported a Goldwater button." Billie pretended to gag.

I told her how David Wilson, the class comedian, chubby in his white shirt, narrow tie, and grey sweater vest, drew the ire of our class by sprouting his conservative views. When the drama teacher saw me with my Goldwater button, she exclaimed: "My goodness, there are two of you!"

"But that is so incompatible with your whole career and your views today," Billie said.

"Yes, that's why by college I turned around completely. I came to realize that the Democrats were more in tune with the civil rights and anti-war movements. I wound up campaigning for Eugene McCarthy and voting absentee for Humphrey in my first election in '68 and then for McGovern in '72. A born again liberal, that's me."

On the Tuesday of the 2000 presidential election, after our therapy session had ended, I suggested that Billie have a glass of wine with us and watch the early returns.

"Okay," she said, "but just one glass." She drank three glasses of wine with us as we watched the returns, and only when we were confident that Gore had won Florida and was on his way to being elected, did my trusty Billie go home.

Despite my early misgivings, I began to look forward to my therapy sessions with Billie, as much for our political discussions as for the regimen that we hoped would help me get better.

12 Old Mosely

Old Mosely is my nickname for the motorized wheelchair that the hospital ordered so I could be mobile. I'd been authorized to work at home based on my medical condition, but this arrangement was not altogether safe. A motorized wheelchair would afford the mobility that would allow me to return to my office. My physical therapy sessions with Billie would continue as before, every Tuesday and Thursday evening at seven. Terri and I would be sure to leave by six on those days so we'd get home in time, even if rush hour traffic was bad. In time, I'd learn to take the metro so she and I wouldn't have to operate like inseparable twins.

Tom, the salesman, and a young woman assisting him drove down from Baltimore a month after my release from the hospital to deliver the chair to my apartment. They stayed long enough to train me on how to maneuver it, which isn't as easy as you think. We took it for a spin in the hallway, and I drove it as carefully as I could at the lowest speed. Still, the toggle was extremely sensitive, and I couldn't keep from zigzagging back and forth in every direction. I was back at the boardwalk at Asbury Park as a little squirt driving bumper cars, first colliding into one wall and then the other. Thank goodness no one else was around, especially little old ladies in their own motorized chairs. After half an hour Tom declared me fit to drive, said a Hail Mary, and left me to my own devices.

Although my new chair seemed fast within the close confines of my apartment, it moved like a tortoise outside. This suited me okay because I planned to use it mainly to go to work and around the neighborhood. For longer excursions, it was easy enough to take along in the car. We bought a metal ramp so that Terri could guide it into our Subaru hatch without needing to break it down into parts, which would have been a royal pain. Guiding it into the hatch took some skill because you had to develop a feel for the toggle, the stick used to steer the chair. Terri became the one person who could accomplish the task comfortably. Even so, in bad weather Old Mosely (a name I chose in a flight of whimsy) skidded on the ramp, making the endeavor even more challenging. Luckily, for several months it never rained or snowed while we loaded and unloaded Old Mosely, even though we were commuting to and from work every day. One day, on our way to the Safeway, the skies opened up just after Terri had rolled Old Mosely into the hatch. Terri expressed concern about guiding the chair down the ramp outdoors in the teeming rain. "It'll skid and I'll get soaked." However, as soon as we pulled up to the store entrance, the rain let up. We began to attribute mystical powers to our new friend.

Another time we went to the movies but had to transport the chair in Terri's Toyota Tercel because the Subaru was in the shop. First I transferred from the chair into the passenger seat, as I was taught to do by the physical therapists in the rehab unit of the hospital. Then Terri broke Old Mosely down into its several parts, and put the parts into the trunk of the car. When we got to the outdoor lot near the movie house, she reconstructed the chair. Voila. Only one problem: now, the toggle was steering it in the wrong direction! When I pushed the toggle to the right Old Mosely would turn left and visa versa. Imagine steering your car left only to have it turn right.

That day the movie was crowded with children who, unbeknownst to their parents or guardians, were placing themselves in harm's way. The auditorium was down one flight, so I attempted to steer toward the elevator. I almost squashed the feet of one little girl who gave me a quizzical look.

Frustrated as hell, I shouted "Damn it, Terri, you steer this for me. I can't."

"Shush, Michael. There are all these kids and their parents. They'll think you're a madman."

"Better than smooshing them. That wouldn't look so hot on my resume, would it? Screw this, it's going all over the place."

Somehow we managed to maneuver the chair into the elevator and, once in the auditorium, we settled for a back row seat. The movie sucked big time, some animated kid's flick and I wasn't enthralled with kids at that moment. I was distracted and anxious about Old Mosely. *What has gone wrong? Is there such a thing as a chair therapist?*

When the movie was over, we waited patiently for everyone else to leave before embarking on the perilous journey back to the parking lot.

When we got to the car, I transferred into the passenger seat and Terri, once again, began to disassemble Old Mosely. As she did this, she realized that in putting the chair back together earlier, she had gotten the wires crossed, so that was why when I'd pressed the toggle to the right the chair would head toward the left. We each breathed a sigh of relief when we found that simply switching the placement of the wires solved Old Mosely's directional dyslexia.

Old Mosely was a good indoor chair because it could turn on a dime. When I returned to the office the week after the chair arrived, I maneuvered it into the elevator, down the hall, through the door to the suite of offices where I worked, into my office, and around to the front of my desk. What fun. There wasn't much maneuvering room behind my desk, however, and one of Old Mosely's flaws was that it didn't truly appreciate its own strength. Sometime in the course of my first week back in the office, I backed up from my desk, forgetting to switch to the lowest speed. Crunch. Old Mosely had smacked the wall behind my desk! Surveying the damage, I was dismayed to see a gaping hole in the wall. The next day I brought in a batik we'd picked up at a street market in Tanzania. It fit nicely on the wall, concealing the hole. I also solicited the help of colleagues to move the desk closer to the center of my office. I was careful after that to keep my chair at low speed, at least until we were in the open hallway. Even so, in my first week or two, I couldn't avoid creating a few scratches and dents on some of the furniture in my office.

A woman in the administrative office named Martha stopped by to discuss devices that I'd need to help me get around the work place. We decided that I could use push buttons on the doors to the office suites so that Old Mosely wouldn't wreck the doors as we tried to enter.

Since I couldn't manage the key to the rest room—no finger muscles—a push button would be necessary there as well. In the meantime, I found useful the urinals of the type provided by the hospital for patients confined to bed. I couldn't afford the luxury of self-consciousness. I opted for the path of least resistance, whatever avenue was most practical and got the job done.

So, I survived at home as well as at the office by making use of these urinals. My work colleagues didn't need to know what I was doing. I brought one into the office contained in a blue coverlet ("the blue thing" as Terri and I referred to it) that we had bought at REI for the Kilimanjaro journey. I placed the blue thing behind my desk on the window ledge. When I needed to use it, I would lock my door, place my "do not disturb" sign outside, and pee into the urinal. At the end of the day, my sainted wife (who, conveniently, worked on another floor in the same building) would empty it and clean it out. No one ever asked what the blue thing was behind my desk, and I never offered.

The push buttons were installed in the suites within a few weeks, but the one for the men's room seemed to be taking forever. I phoned the administrative office to ask about the status of the rest room push button. "Oh, the men should be around to install it later in the week," Martha explained.

"That's good," I said, "I'm getting a little tired of holding it in."

Each floor of the garage where we parked had wheelchair access by way of a ramp or cut curb leading to the elevator entrance. Otherwise, Old Mosely wouldn't have been able to navigate the steep step up to the entrance. We usually stopped by the elevators first to allow me room to transfer from the car into Old Mosely. Then Terri would find a space to park. On rare occasions, when it was time to go home, we'd find that someone had squeezed a car into a nonexistent space, blocking access to the ramp. I'd have to roll to another level where I could access the entrance, and Terri would pick me up in our car. Our only recourse was to leave a caustic note. I don't know what I'd have done if I were alone and there was only one floor with wheelchair access. Like the man named Charley, who in the well-known ballad, "rode forever 'neath the streets of Boston," I'd be "the man who never returned."

In addition to being relatively slow (even at its fastest speed, Old Mosely's pace was that of a brisk walk), the chair couldn't go far, even on a full charge. At the end of a typical workday, which involved rolling in and out of garages and around the office complex, one or two blinking lights would pop up on the toggle arm, which meant its battery was getting low. Time to charge it. If we wanted to catch a movie at the *Uptown,* about a mile down Connecticut Avenue, we could make the round trip on foot, but that was about the farthest we could chance taking Old Mosely without the car. Since I was petrified of getting stuck somewhere with a dead battery, we made it a habit to charge Old Mosely every night at bedtime.

"Terri, don't forget my water. Did you check the front door lock? Turn out the lights? Remember to charge Old Mosely? Okay, good night then."

Terri, Billie and Old Mosely, working together to weave a safety net for me until the day I could walk again.

13 Some Medical Complications, A High School Graduation, and the Challenge of Flying

Even before Old Mosely arrived on the scene, I'd re-entered the hospital twice due to blood clotting in my leg, culminating in a pulmonary embolism. These events were a direct result of my immobility. At home, I was now receiving monthly treatments of Cytoxan, a chemotherapy generally reserved for cancer patients, albeit at a lower dose. My treatments were intended to suppress my pesky immune system in order to halt its unwelcome attack on my peripheral nerves.

When I'd suffered the symptoms of my first pulmonary embolism in mid-May, I'd no idea what was happening. Because of the Cytoxan treatments, Dr. Sherman had assumed that I'd come down with pneumonia, always a risk with a suppressed immune system. An X-ray had confirmed his suspicions, or so he'd thought. The medication he'd prescribed didn't seem to help though, and the pain on my left side kept getting worse. Terri and I had planned to celebrate our wedding anniversary that week by going to a restaurant downtown. But, since I wasn't feeling well and was in no condition to go out on the town, Jane told us to come to her house in Cleveland Park to celebrate instead.

Terri pushed me along in my wheelchair for the five or so blocks to Jane's house, through the alley to the back entrance. I could only enter Jane's house from the rear, since the front entrance had a series of steep steps. We opened the gate and squeezed through a narrow pathway leading to the back courtyard. Rose petals strewn along the way led us to the flagstone patio and the round patio table beautifully set with floating candles, nibbles, wine glasses, and an opened bottle of pinot grigio. That is Jane for you, conjuring up a romantic setting for us. We were moved by her thoughtfulness and generosity. The evening was perfect for alfresco dining, with clear skies and a warm breeze. What better way to celebrate our anniversary? No four-star restaurant could have matched it.

I'd give anything to go back and relive that evening in good health, but it was my misfortune to have been in great discomfort then. At home that night, in bed, I couldn't move or sit up without experiencing severe side pain. Just reaching for my water glass was an ordeal. Terri called Dr. Sherman and left a message. He called back within five minutes. "Take him to the emergency room at GW right away," he said.

Terri called an ambulance, as I found it impossible to transfer into my wheelchair. It was midnight or later by the time we got to the emergency room. The doctors quickly diagnosed a pulmonary embolism. They gave me Percocet for pain and administered an IV of heparin as a fast working blood thinner to break down the clot. I felt much better in a matter of hours. But there I was, back at the hospital. *Is there no end to all of this,* I wanted to shout. It was all I could do to keep from giving up.

I recalled one of the neurologists at the hospital during my first stay assuring me that CIDP was not life threatening. Clearly, he wasn't considering the secondary conditions that can arise because of it. Thrombosis is the clotting of blood within an artery or vein. Encouraged by inflammation and stagnation of blood flow through inactivity, it poses a deadly risk. What can happen is that a clot breaks off and, carried with the flow of blood, lodges in the lungs—a pulmonary embolism. A pulmonary embolism can kill because it has the potential to choke the flow of blood to the brain and cause a stroke. Fortunately, I first came to this knowledge later on when I got home. By then I was out of the woods.

Within a day or two, the heparin had done its job so Dr. Sherman started me on Coumadin, a blood thinner, to help prevent formation of future clots and reduce the risk of repeat episodes. Getting the dosage right, however, can be a tricky business.

The nutritionists at the hospital advised me not to alter my diet significantly and to stay away from certain foods rich in vitamin K, such as leafy vegetables. Vitamin K is known to alter the metabolism of Coumadin, interfering with its effects. Drinking too much alcohol has a similar effect, but I didn't want to give up the precious glasses of Chardonnay that I enjoy evenings, before and with dinner. Thankfully, the doctors I polled were sympathetic and agreed I could keep the habit if I limited myself to no more than two drinks a day.

But I felt weakened from the whole ordeal, if it was even possible to feel weaker than I already did. A tech aide wheeled me to a room where I was to be tested to determine the origin of the clot. The tech left me in the hands of two young female nurses who were ready to conduct the test.

"Do you need help getting up onto the table?"

"I need you two to lift me, actually," I said. "I have CIDP, which means my muscles aren't working and I'm very weak, right now."

"Okay. Let me give you a hand. Try to help as much as you can." I helped as much as I could, like a baby helping its mama change its diapers.

"Boy, you really are a weak Willy."

"Yes, I know. I'm sorry." Together, they managed to lift and drag me onto the table and proceeded to conduct the exam. Then they called the muscular nurses' assistant who helped get me back into the chair and wheeled me back to my room. It was then that I got mad. *Why should I have to apologize for my condition?*

Later that afternoon Terri came over, and a little while later Dr. Richardson stopped by. I complained bitterly to him about how weak I felt, and said that I was worried I was getting worse. He assured me that my weakened state was not due to any relapse in the CIDP, but rather to the ordeal of having suffered through a pulmonary embolism.

Dr. Richardson said that it was about time for my second Cytoxan treatment and that as long as I was back at the hospital for a few days they'd work that into my schedule. He said that they'd start the hydration in preparation for the treatment that evening.

"This means that you will have to urinate all night long," he warned. "At first, the color of your urine will be yellow but by the second or third time it will be pale and, eventually clear as water." When he finished explaining the drill he left.

After he went out, Terri turned to me. "I'm beginning to like him," she said.

"Yes," I said. "If he'll take all that time to dwell on the changing color of my urine, he must have a human side, after all."

During my lengthy stay at GW the previous month, I was intensely focused on the treatments, therapy sessions, and the constant attention of doctors and nurses, too busy to obsess about my misfortune. In my mind, I was destined to get better even if it might take longer than we'd first hoped. Therefore, I believed it counter-productive to feel sorry for myself, to ask "why me?" But now I was weaker and feeling quite hopeless. The uncertainty of whether I'd ever recover was weighing on me. The days were still filled with activity, but at night, when the therapists had gone home, the nurses and doctors had each done their thing, and the visitors had drifted away, I could hear myself asking "why me, why is this now happening to me?"

I confided my thoughts to a nurses' aide I'd come to like and trust. "It's all right to ask "why me?" she said, as she helped move me up on the bed. "You'll find no good answers, but it's okay to ask."

They kept me at the hospital for several days to ensure that the Coumadin they were prescribing was the right dose. When I came home it was almost June, time for Terri and me to cement our plans for Jessica's high school graduation party that Jane would host. Jane's house just down the street would make for a much better venue than our apartment.

Lots of folks came to celebrate and cheer Jessica the evening of her graduation. She had earned this bash, having overcome serious learning disabilities, the separation and divorce of her parents, and the subsequent death of her mom. It was especially good to see Allison, Jessica's best friend from Ivymount. It had been several years since they'd seen each other. Allison had always needed a wheelchair due to a deformity of her spine. When her folks wheeled her into Jane's backyard, they expressed shock to find me in a wheelchair as well. I gave them the short version.

In addition to our close friends and relatives in the D.C. area, a few people came from afar. Patsy and Judy drove down from their safe havens in Manhattan. This was the first time I'd seen them since the onset of my illness. Patsy and her husband Danny had wanted to visit when I was in the hospital. "We're coming right down," Patsy told Terri. "Judy too." But I told them to wait for Jessica's graduation, which was then less than two months away.

"Okay, we'll definitely be there. By the way," Patsy added, "Judy has a theory on you. She thinks you've used up your mobility. She thinks everyone in the world has only so much mobility and you've used all of yours up with all that running stuff and mountain climbing, which explains your neuropathy." This from my sedentary extended family, each of whom would groan if they had to walk a city block. I laughed.

Arthur also drove south from his home in Maplewood, New Jersey. As a youngster, Arthur was brilliant and witty and, I must add, something of a wise guy. He excelled at just about anything he took up, whether bowling, pool, or golf. We saw each other mostly during summers on the Jersey shore where his folks and mine owned second homes. He also shared my family's summertime affection for thoroughbred racing.

Being in Arthur's company was always an adventure. I recall the time he insisted on my going for a ride with him on the back of his new motorcycle. We didn't make it past his driveway before tipping over at the underwhelming speed of one mile per hour. And then there was the time when, at age sixteen, I drove a golf cart into the water trying to make it over a footbridge. My mistake. I thought he'd pointed to the footbridge instead of the other, wider bridge meant for carts. I remember him jumping from the cart as soon as he recognized my error. Valiantly, I stuck with the cart all the way, tipping over and sliding into the creek. "That took imagination, determination, courage, and stupidity," he said later in the day, as he recounted our misadventure to our families.

Tragically, both of Arthur's parents succumbed to cancer when he was around sixteen. He spent much of his youth trying to find himself, exploring various ventures, including investing in a small stable of racehorses. In this way, he managed to fritter away much of his substantial inheritance. Eventually he met and married Liz, a community college teacher who lived in Maplewood, and who was about fifteen years his senior. Liz became his salvation. With Liz, he settled down and took a teaching position at the same college where she taught.

Arthur and Liz came to visit Jessica and me in Washington many times over the years. Their trips became more frequent after I had ended my marriage to Sylvia, and they felt safe from being tossed out of the house. Their visits were an excuse for me to become a tourist in my own town. We traipsed around the mall, exploring the Smithsonian museums, the National Gallery of Art, and the monuments. They particularly enjoyed excursions to Mount Vernon over the holiday season and Hillwood Museum and Gardens, the former home of Marjorie Merriweather Post. Hillwood, which is on a quiet cul-de-sac in the Cleveland Park neighborhood, just a mile or so from my apartment house, is a gem of a museum that now houses Ms. Post's collection of Russian art and objects. It is a well-kept secret in Washington.

When I married Terri, Arthur came to D.C. with Liz to serve as my best man. Patsy, Judy and Arthur all expressed gratitude that I'd found a sane, sensible and devoted wife in Terri. Arthur and Liz continued to visit Terri and me in Washington, just as we would see them whenever we went to New York.

But Arthur came alone to Jessica's graduation. Sadly, Liz had died of a stroke in early April, just one week before my lengthy hospitalization. Notwithstanding my growing health problems, Terri, Jessica and I had made the trip to Maplewood for the memorial service. Terri drove most of the way up. I took the wheel for the return trip that evening amidst a severe rainstorm. Little did I know then that it would be my last chance to drive for several years, and my last time driving without hand controls.

Midway through the graduation party, Terri announced a toast to the new graduate. We watched Jessica open gifts that included a shoebox filled with 100 one-dollar bills. Someone poured a glass with champagne and handed it to me. I took it with both hands. In order to do a proper toast, I shifted the glass to my left hand and raised it chin level. That was the best I could do without my wrist flopping over and the champagne spilling out. Patsy, splendid in her gray designer suit, pretended not to notice. Judy snapped photos, while Arthur looked on.

The next day Jessica would leave with her classmates for a school-sponsored one-week graduation trip to Jamaica, another well-earned treat. In the fall, she'd begin a two-year vocational program at Lesley College in Cambridge, Massachusetts. I pledged to take her to Boston in September whether or not I got back some of the mobility I'd apparently used up.

When the time came for Jessica to return from her graduation trip, Terri and I met her at the airport. As we were waiting for her at the gate, I started coughing for no apparent reason. I guessed that either I was having another pulmonary embolism or the old one was flaring up. I went for an X-ray the next morning and back to the emergency room later that day.

I didn't have nearly as much pain with my second episode, probably because I was able to tell what was happening and get to the emergency room quickly. The doctors there thought this episode might simply be a recurrence of the first one. My blood was still not thin enough—so they'd once again have to fiddle with the dosage. I was again given an IV of heparin and my third monthly Cytoxan treatment was scheduled. Terri wasn't amused. It seemed an eternity before a room was ready for me. Once again we were faced with an all-nighter at the emergency room resting on uncomfortable cots or chairs.

After I'd been released from the hospital following the first occurrence, nurses had come to my home from time to time to draw blood. Now it was decided, just to be safe, that I'd go down to Dr. Sherman's office three times a week to do these blood draws until we could be confident that we had the dosage right and my blood numbers remained consistently at a therapeutic level. This meant, of course, that Terri would have to take time off from work to drive me to Dr. Sherman's office on K Street and back home. By now my motorized chair had been delivered. Three times a week we'd load Old Mosely into the Subaru hatch, park at the GW garage, roll to the doctor's office, and then return home. Then she'd leave for work.

On the Friday after I returned home from the hospital, following my second bout with a pulmonary embolism, we went out to dinner with Jane and Janet (another work friend). Janet had worked at Torts with Jane and me for many years, but had quit about a year before to engage in legal work overseas. Janet had also been in the wedding party when I married Terri. So we were going out to dine with close friends—family you might say. And I wasn't on my best behavior.

We chose a good Thai restaurant on Wisconsin Avenue in Cleveland Park. I'd promised Terri that I'd forego wine at least until we could be confident that the medication was working as it should. We didn't really know whether wine played any role at all in my last episode, but we weren't taking any chances. I'd faithfully stopped drinking at home. But now the women ordered a bottle of white wine with dinner and I was sorely tempted.

"Let me just have a sip of yours, Terri."

"Okay, one sip," she said as I tried to hold the glass. But I wasn't managing to grip the glass very well. Terri took the glass from me and held it to my lips tilting it so that I could drink. But she tilted it a bit too much. I started coughing and some of the wine spilled down my shirt.

"Just let me hold the glass, or let me pour my own," I said, raising my voice. Jane and Janet looked on amused, and maybe a little uncomfortable.

"No, Michael. You promised not to drink more than a sip. Let's just have a nice evening with Jane and Janet."

"Well then give me your glass to hold myself. I can't drink it when you're pouring it down my throat," I said. I was like a toddler, whining and pouting because his favorite toy had been taken away.

Terri gave me the glass and I took a healthy sip and then another. And another. Finally, she snatched the glass and placed it out of my reach. Janet changed the conversation to other things, while I pouted. Terri didn't say a word the rest of dinner.

After dinner, we paid the bill and Terri stormed down the street. I caught up with her at the light. She was crying.

"What's wrong," I asked, knowing full well what was wrong.

"You know, it's not all about you," she said. "I've had to get up in the middle of the night to take you to the ER and try to sleep in a chair while you're lying down on a cot, waiting to transfer to a room. Do you I think that I enjoy these little trips to the ER? Do you think I want to keep doing this? And it's me that has to drive you to Dr. Sherman's office three times a week. But all you think about is your wine. Your precious wine."

"I'm sorry," I said.

"No, that's not good enough. Let's just go home."

We dropped Jane and Janet off and then Terri drove home. As is usually the case when we've had a spat, I said I was sorry a half dozen times. I've never been a moody person. I'm not one to hold my anger inside for long. If some small thing makes me upset I blow up and within minutes I become remorseful. Terri had learned that about me, at times the hard way.

"Tell me you were wrong," she insisted.

"I was wrong." The words every spouse longs to hear.

"Very wrong."

"I was very wrong."

"And you'll behave better and lay off the wine, at least for now."

"I promise." She studied my face.

"Give me a hug." We hugged.

"I love you," I said.

"I love you too." Now, her crying was mixed with laughter.

It dawned on me how much Terri had to put up with, and how lucky I was.

I took my first airplane trip in a wheelchair in September 2000. That's when Terri and I took Jessica to Cambridge, just across the Charles River from Boston, to begin her two-year vocational program at Lesley College. It was the first of several trips we would take over the next couple of years, always with logistical challenges.

After much thought and discussion, we opted not to take Old Mosely because we didn't want to risk damaging or losing any of its parts in transit. Instead, we took my manual wheelchair. We also took other essential paraphernalia: my walker, my safety belt, some of the lighter weights I used for physical therapy, and a urinal. This seemed much like traveling with Jessica when she was an infant, when her mom and I would take along a stroller, snuggly, basinet, car seat, and diaper bag.

I could use my walker for exercise in the hotel corridors as long as Terri accompanied me while holding my safety belt. She couldn't prevent me from falling, but she could soften my fall if she was quick to act. We'd become compulsive about my doing some physical therapy every day, so the weights came too. And, of course, we took the urinal discreetly hidden in the same blue REI sack we'd used on the Kilimanjaro climb. This I could not do without. Because I couldn't rise up from my chair under my own steam, I couldn't use the facilities anywhere, any place. So we took the urinal whenever we went out.

We notified the airlines well in advance that I'd need assistance in getting on and off the plane with the tiny wheelchair the airlines reserve for such endeavors. At each boarding, the attendants strapped me in tight, asked me to keep my hands on my lap, carried me down the aisle, and lifted me out of the chair and into my seat. Terri followed close behind. On this and later trips, we were usually the first to board and the last to get off. On one trip, however, I had to wait for the airlines to come up with a chair, and was carried onto the airplane last, in full view of all the passengers. Like Quasimodo, the hunchback of Notre Dame, being carried through the streets of Paris as the Pope of Fools, I became the center of unwanted attention, the freak in a circus sideshow. I kept my eyes down to avoid the inevitable stares. We eventually received an apology from the airlines.

During this first trip to Boston I felt like I'd left behind what little independence remained to me. Terri and Jessica took turns pushing me around in my chair wherever we went. Bumpity bump, bumpity bump along the cobblestone streets of old Cambridge, up and down curbs, street to sidewalk. Like European cities built centuries ago, the historic parts of Boston have few cut curbs and the quaint cobblestone streets, while picturesque, are not exactly wheelchair friendly. I wondered what folks with similar disabilities did in days of yore. Maybe they were hidden away in back rooms or attics, cared for by loved ones if they were lucky. It was some consolation, I supposed, that I wasn't enduring my illness in the seventeenth century.

Crockett House, a three-story wood frame house, was one of several the college used for students. Jessica's room was on the third floor. That meant I'd have to wait outside while Terri helped move her in. Terri took a Polaroid photo for my sake. A simple room for Jessica and her one roommate. I could see she'd already fastened photos of us, her boyfriend, and our cat, Zoey, to a bulletin board above her desk.

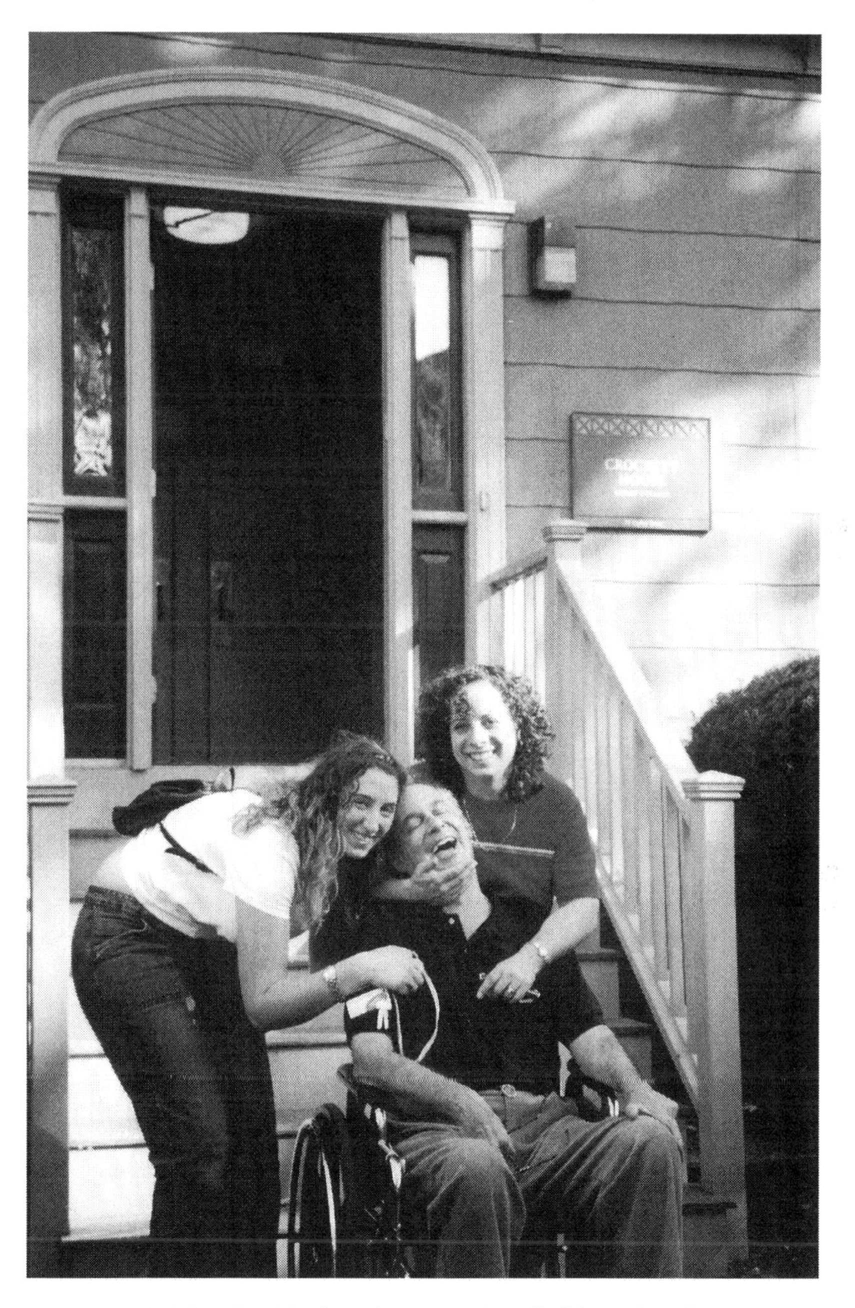

Michael with daughter Jessica (left) and wife
Terri (right) at Crockett House, Fall 2000

The following month when we flew to Boston for parents weekend, I got to see my daughter's room for real. I relive this moment with fond memories from time to time:

We arrive early afternoon and Jessica is waiting for us outside with her roommate, Abbey, and Abbey's family. Jessica introduces us. Terri says we should all walk to the main square for a bite to eat, that there is no need to go upstairs to the room since it is small and I'd already seen the photo. Realizing that I hadn't yet seen the room in person, Abbey's dad and brother insist on carrying me up. They don't take no for an answer. Dressed in jeans and t-shirts, they lift me in my chair and carry me up several steps to the porch and inside through the front door, the dad taking up the front, the brother behind me. The staircase is narrow, too narrow I think. This will never work. But somehow it does. Huffing and puffing, they lift me high above the banisters, the only way they could navigate these steps. They are lifting me so high I could touch the ceiling if I wanted. As they clamber past the first level, the girls who live in the house and other visiting parents pop out of their rooms and start to cheer. When we get to Jessica's room, Abbey's dad puts me down gently. Boy, is he strong. The room is just like the photo, but I'm glad to actually see it for myself. Once they've carried me back down to the street, we all stroll to the square for lunch. My treat.

On yet another trip to Boston, we rented a motorized chair. This chair resembled a normal wheelchair, only with a souped-up motor attached to it. This chair was fun in a perverse sort of way. Unlike Old Mosely's relatively smooth, slow gait, this rental zipped along at a fast pace with a herky-jerky motion. We traversed Harvard Square, turned along Massachusetts Avenue, Cambridge's main street, past mimes performing for the crowds, past newsstands, past the Harvard Coop. Folks leaped out of the way as I zigzagged about. Now I was assuming command, asserting my independence. I enjoyed this excursion far more than the last two trips, when I'd been pushed about like so much cargo. Never before, I would later brag to my friends and colleagues, had I had so many lovely young coeds falling head over heels just for me.

Our first cross-country adventure came the following summer when Terri scheduled a flight to Seattle for an appellate argument in one of her immigration cases. Since Seattle was where her mother and sister lived, I tagged along to join in the family visit. Luckily, we had a row of seats on the airplane to ourselves. As this was my first cross-country flight since my illness—indeed, my first flight over two hours—I'd never before had to think about how on earth I'd make my way to the toilet in the front or back of the plane. Since I still needed to be carried onto the aircraft strapped into one of those tiny chairs, I envisioned no practical means by which I could use the facilities.

What do wheelchair bound people do when they need to use the facilities, I wondered. Growing up, I was painfully self-conscious, always worried about what others would think if in the course of some undertaking I looked awkward or un-cool. Over time, I came to realize that self-consciousness is an indulgence that must yield in the face of struggle. On Kilimanjaro, whether climbing uphill over large rocks or down the mountain along a steep pebbly trail, I had no choice but to traverse the course on hands and knees or butt first, even as youngsters half my age loped along without a care, as if they were kids playing hop scotch.

So now, with a row of seats to ourselves, I'd have little choice but to discreetly use the urinal we carried in the blue REI coverlet, combined with one of the small blankets available on the plane. I had fretted for days over the prospect of how to make this work without anyone noticing. When the day of travel arrived, I wore shorts to facilitate the process. Nothing could be more awkward or un-cool. But as with the mountain climb, this was no time for self-consciousness.

We stayed in a downtown hotel the night before Terri's argument. Seattle is a hilly city, not like San Francisco, of course, but still there are a lot of steep ups and downs. We used my own manual wheelchair for this trip. On our first afternoon, Terri pushed me up and down the hills to do a little exploring before dinner. We rolled down a steep hill to Pike's Market and watched as the fishmongers in white coats tossed the fish back and forth for the benefit of the tourists. We bought hot pepper jelly at a boutique along the way. Then Terri pushed me back up the hill and down another. This little jaunt turned out to be challenging exercise for her, but as usual, my sainted wife took it in stride. I hid my guilt stoically.

That evening, we settled on a small intimate Italian bistro for dinner. This place was at the bottom of a hill, not too far from Pike's Market and Puget Sound. Terri was already well prepared for her ten-minute argument, so we relaxed, sharing a bottle of Soave Bolla with our meal. It was after dinner that trouble found us. If you think it's hard work for a small woman to push a 180-pound man up a steep hill in a wheelchair, you might try it after drinking a bottle of wine accompanied by fine Italian cooking. Chug, chug, sweat, curse, groan. She stopped several times along what had to be the longest block in any city anywhere.

"You made it up Kilimanjaro," I said. "So this should be easy."

She wondered out loud whether she might just give up and see how well I could roll backwards to the bottom, where we could call for a cab.

"I'll buy you a nightcap back at the hotel," I bargained.

Just then, when it seemed that Terri had reached the limits of her endurance, we spied a young couple with a baby carriage headed downhill. They instantly recognized our dilemma and came to the rescue. The man, in his early thirties, dressed in a polo shirt and sports coat, took charge of the chair and completed the climb as easily as taking a Sunday stroll in the park.

Home free, I would live to fight another day.

I bought us each a gin and tonic when we were back within the safe confines of our hotel.

After Terri's court appearance, we spent an extended weekend visiting with her mother, Eleanor, her sister, Lara, Lara's husband, Maurice, and their little boy, Cameron.

Eleanor lived in an apartment complex that had a swimming pool. I sat in my wheelchair by the edge of the pool under the hot sun, wishing I could jump in to cool off.

"I could help you get in, but we'd need a rescue squad to get you out," Terri said. "How about if I splash you?"

"Okay," I said, settling for repeated splashes.

Sunday, we went with Lara and Cameron to a small beach on the north shore of Lake Washington, near Lara's home. Terri pushed my chair onto the sand where I watched with envy as Cameron splashed about among the other kids at the beach. I loved lake swimming. I'd swum in Lake Washington a few years back when Terri and I had first gotten engaged. I knew that once in the water, I could swim, or at least, float for a good long while; however, getting in and out of the lake was the problem. If only the world were flooded with water, I'd exist on an even playing field.

On Monday we packed for the long plane ride home. I wore shorts again. This time, we didn't have the whole row to ourselves. A middle-aged woman sat on the aisle. Terri took the middle seat while I sat by the window. When, midway through the flight, I needed to pee, I looked all around. The woman on the aisle was intently focused on her book. The flight attendants were occupied elsewhere. No one was walking in the aisle. In tribute to paranoia, I even looked out the window to make sure no one was peering in from outside. Confident that the coast was clear, I placed the blanket over my legs. Terri handed me the urinal in the blue REI sack. I removed the urinal and discreetly slid it under the blanket. The noise of the aircraft drowned out any sound from my effort.

14 Christmas In New York

The winter holidays, from late December 2000 thru January 2001, not only failed to bring any sign of recovery, but the events that unfolded then may have set me back, complicating any potential healing. We'd planned to spend Christmas week in Manhattan visiting Patsy, Judy, and Aunt Ceal. Ceal was nearing 90 by then and showing signs of dementia.

On the day of my office Christmas party, two days before our planned trip, I stumbled while walking with my walker. I simply misplaced one of my feet, but I went down hard and sprained my ankle rather badly. My colleagues helped me up and placed an ice pack on the injured foot, which I kept on until party time. The next morning the ankle was swollen and discolored, so Terri drove me to my doctor's office. The nurses devised a little splint for support. There seemed no reason to put off the trip; I'd just have to do as little walking as possible. Terri drove Jessica and me to the city with me stretched out in the back seat, my foot elevated for the entire trip.

Normally in New York we would stay with Terri's Aunt Julia in Gramercy, but she was inundated with work, so we booked a wheelchair accessible room at the Hotel Emerson at Broadway and 63rd Street, near Lincoln Center and not far from Aunt Ceal's or Patsy's apartments. The Emerson was an old, refurbished hotel. I had stayed there before several times while on official business for the government.

Although the room we'd booked was said to be accessible, the tiny bathroom wasn't. We worked it out that I'd motor over to the bathroom door and Terri would help me up and into my walker. Then I would limp sideways to where she could help me step into the tub. Less than ideal but doable. The bellman brought a chair for the tub.

Lying in bed that night, I could feel a sensation of numbness creeping up both my legs, almost to the knees. I feared a relapse. Relapses can occur in CIDP patients, especially during the first year. I was now nine months into my illness, if I counted from the time of my first hospitalization. I chose to begin counting then rather than from my first signs of illness several months earlier. That way I could stretch out the 18-month recovery time I supposedly had if I was to get better. That was my psychology. Not getting better was the primary demon haunting my dreams at night. It was the most frightening thought I could have and one that I pushed aside during the day. I was working too hard not to get better.

I knew that relapses were more likely to occur in CIDP patients who suffered trauma. My sprained ankle provided sufficient reason for me to suspect a relapse. Since I was still seeing Dr. Richardson periodically, I resolved to make an urgent appointment with him when I got home.

I found the trip to New York a misery. The trip marked my first winter with neuropathy. Captive to the wheelchair, there was no way I could build up the body heat needed to mitigate the effects of the bitter winter winds. For me, this had to be the coldest Christmas ever. I can't say exactly what the temperature was, but taking into account the wheelchair factor, it had to be below zero.

On the day before Christmas the three of us went to see a movie at a theater near the hotel. We were to be at Ceal's for dinner by six so we had time to spare. At least a theater would provide warmth and comfort, even if the movie were a dud. I didn't own any gloves that I could get my hands and fingers into without a struggle, so we first stopped at a shop on Broadway. I bought the sorriest looking pale green mittens. "Those are girl's mittens, Dad," Jessica said.

"Beggars can't be choosers, Jessica," Terri said. "At least I can coax his hands into them easily enough."

One problem, however. I couldn't handle the joystick to steer Old Mosely, so I had to remove my right mitten. "Grin n' bear it," I sighed. We bought the movie tickets and realized we had over an hour to waste before the film was to begin. Nothing to do but walk around outside, in the frigid air.

I had grown up on the west side, so I led my family a few blocks up Broadway to 72nd street. I wanted to search for the old Royal Bakery on 72nd, just west of Broadway. It was there that I used to go to pick up bagels for brunch after Sunday school. While bagels had been my main mission, I'd also treat myself to jelly tarts and black n' white cookies. The tarts were the best anywhere, with chunks of almonds galore and powdered sugar with raspberry or apricot filling. The black and white cookies, although common enough, were also like none other.

So we crossed Broadway past the bustling subway station that dominates the island where Broadway crosses Amsterdam, and headed west on 72nd street. We combed the north side of the street all the way to West End Avenue, but no bakery. The Royal must have closed or moved. So many of the old shops and delis were still there, but not the Royal. How disappointing. "We still have time before the movie," I said, by way of consolation. "Let's duck into the deli across the street and warm ourselves with hot chocolate."

"Great idea, Dad," Jessica said. By now my toes were as frozen as icicles. We were all shivering.

After the movie we went back to the hotel to nap and change for dinner. Try as I might, I couldn't get my hands or feet to warm up. I snuggled under the blankets. Terri brought me a hot washcloth. No dice. Poor circulation was a by-product of my neuropathy. It would be a long winter.

When it was time for dinner we drove the mile or so north to Ceal's apartment. Normally, I'd have insisted on walking up Broadway to 81st Street, and one block over to her building on West End Avenue. This walk is memory lane for me, past what used to be the Beacon movie house where as a little tike I had coaxed my grandmother into taking me to see *Godzilla* four times. Past the Broadway Fruit and Nut Shop which has stayed in place seemingly forever. Past H&H Bagels and Zabar's, where I used to go for the Nova Scotia lox in the days before it expanded to three times its original size. So many food shops to choose from around Broadway in the 70s and 80s. What did the folks across the park on the east side do for food, I always wondered.

But now it was too cold to walk and Old Mosely didn't have a full charge, so we took the car. Ceal's place was a small, smoky one-bedroom affair, quite a contrast to the eleven-room apartment we'd all shared when I was a kid. Jessica and I used to stay with Ceal on our visits to New York before I met Terri, but her place was too cramped for all of us and, in any event, staying with Ceal was no joy. She smoked like a chimney and shut all of the windows. Just having dinner there was stifling enough.

Patsy and Danny lived with their three White Highland terriers two blocks away from Ceal in a one-bedroom at Broadway and 83rd Street. Judy was holed up with her dogs in a studio apartment on the east side that she has rented since graduating college. So, on this trip, staying at the Emerson worked best for us.

When we arrived at Ceal's, Patsy, Danny, and Judy were already there, as were several guests. As I rolled in, Ceal turned to Patsy and asked "What happened to him?"

Ceal was dressed in a pants suit. Her orange bouffant had been freshened recently. Weekly trips to her hairdresser were now her sole outdoor excursions. Otherwise, she occupied herself with mystery novels, radio talk shows, and cigarettes. I gave Aunt Ceal a kiss and explained my condition to her. "What happened to you?" she repeated in her gravelly voice after I finished my explanation. The short-term memory seemed to be running on empty. She put out a cigarette and lit another.

"If you're going to keep puffing away, Mamu, I'm going to have to open the windows," Judy said. Ceal frowned and looked at me as if to ask "what am I to do?"

Ceal had smoked all her life. I imagined her lighting up as she emerged from the womb. One time, years earlier, when she was having medical issues of some sort, Patsy begged her to quit smoking. "Ma, at least cut down on the number of packs a day you smoke."

"What d'ya want me to do, masturbate?" was Ceal's response. Nonetheless, going on 90, she seemed the perfect poster gal for the tobacco industry.

Now Ceal turned to Terri. "What happened to him?" she asked in a hushed voice, pointing at me.

When I was a youngster, Aunt Ceal was like a second mother to me. While my mother ran the office during the week at Uncle Lou's Brooklyn factory, it was Ceal, together with my grandmother, who watched over us. During summers on the Jersey shore she'd take us to the boardwalk at Asbury Park, or bowling, or to the movies. Arthur would sometimes come along. I recall the Paramount Theater on the boardwalk, an enormous brick building with high ceilings that had fake clouds always in motion. I had a hard time sitting still for double features and often found myself gazing up at the fake clouds. Later on, Ceal or Patsy would explain the plot to me. Judy had no patience.

Every Friday, early in the evening, we'd pile in the car for the short ride to the Elberon train station where we'd pick up my mother and Uncle Lou, who were arriving for the weekend. On Saturdays, the adults regularly went to the horse races at Monmouth Park. For a time I collected their losing tickets but by age 13 I was going too.

I became a racing addict, in large part due to my family's summertime affection for the sport. I recall the days when we'd pile into the car after dinner and drive to the news store by the Elberon train station, in order to pick up the three racing papers that our family had reserved—one for Pop, one for Sis, and one for Aunt Ceal. The racing form is every true horseplayer's bible. It contains detailed past performances of every horse entered in every race at all the major racetracks in the country. This was no time for sharing. I once tried to steal a quick look at Pop's paper when he was snoozing. "Who took my paper," he grumped. Well, I'd *thought* he was snoozing.

Sis, Pop, and Aunt Ceal would spend the remainder of the evening figuring the horses for the next day based on past performances detailed in the racing form. This endeavor could be a near science, depending on how obsessed one was. Aunt Ceal proved to be the most ardent student in our family. Using a slide rule and statistics from the racing paper, she'd assign numerical values to each horse entered in every race at Monmouth Park. She was quite good at it, and I always thought she could be a professional race tout. If she had only stuck to her own predictions, she might have won a lot of money, but like many hopeful betters she preferred to put her two dollars on a long shot. My mother, on the other hand, paid lip service to the task. She'd study the horses for a brief time, but then she'd quickly turn to perusing other news in the paper, or she'd return to her book. My family often joked about the time when my mother remarked on two candidates running for state office. "Lefkowitz and O'Toole are neck and neck," she said. Aunt Ceal looked up, puzzled. "Fran, what are you talking about? Are these horses to watch? I don't see either a Lefkowitz or O'Toole entered at Monmouth Park?" It might be aptly said that Aunt Ceal had a one-track mind.

The great racehorse, Kelso, came on the scene just as I began to follow the family tradition and become a student of the sport. He inspired me by his stunning come-from- behind performances. Others of my age would marvel at the feats of Willie Mays, Mickey Mantle, and Y.A. Tittle. Kelso became my sports hero. My fellow high school students saw fit to include the following inscription in my write-up in our senior yearbook: "horse racing is in Mike's blood, and at this very moment Kelso is rounding the bend at his left artery."

Arthur, more than my cousins, immersed himself in my family's summer pastime. He was a constant fixture at the racetrack, in his tweed jacket, sweater vest, and cap. We followed the stakes races all year round and talked horses endlessly. Arthur loved to gamble and was especially adept at numbers. I was in awe of his ability to calculate in his head exactly what a horse would pay on a two dollar bet just by seeing what the tote board showed was the dollar amount bet on the horse.

Before dinner, I tested Ceal's memory of those long ago days. "What was our box number at Monmouth Park," I asked.

"Eighty-eight," she answered. Her long-term memory was still very much intact. Following a few rounds of drinks with cheese and crackers, we sat down to dinner. I rolled over to the head of the extended table in the living area, as that was the only place Old Mosely could fit. We dined on London broil, roast potatoes, and string beans with mushrooms. After dinner, we exchanged the neatly wrapped gifts that had been arranged on and around the card table in the corner. We left when it became clear that Ceal was ready for bed.

"You have to come see us in South Hampton this summer," Patsy said to Terri and me on our way out the door. "You haven't been out in a couple of years. You must see our new addition."

"I'll see how I'm doing," I said. "I'd want to be mobile enough to enjoy your pool and the beach. If not this summer, maybe the next."

We spent several days in the city visiting family, seeing movies, doing brunch on Christmas day, and meeting Julia for dinner. The family visits were fine, but by the end of our stay I was more than ready to return to the comforts of home.

My neurologist didn't need to see me to put me back on prednisone. I'd been off it for several months; now I'd start up again. Thirty milligrams every other day.

Billie suspended walking and climbing stairs to allow time for my ankle to heal. She brought in a machine to apply heat to the ankle that helped speed up the mending process. In the months ahead, I'd explain to her that I felt stronger on prednisone days. On the days I took the medicine I could get up from Old Mosely into my walker on my own. On the other days, I'd need a boost or do it from the lift chair. My walking also seemed steadier on prednisone days. Billie was skeptical. "It's psychological," she'd say.

In January, Terri suggested I take up swim therapy. Sessions were being offered at a county pool in Rockville once a week. I agreed; why not try everything to arouse my dormant muscles? So we went to the pool twice a week; once for therapy one evening a week and once on the weekend to splash around.

The pool complex was large. The therapy took place in a small pool in a separate area from the two Olympic-size pools. Megan, our young therapist, faced a special challenge with me: how to get me in and out of the pool. A long ramp led into the shallow end of the pool, but I couldn't take my chair or walker into the pool. Terri volunteered to stand in for my walker. As we entered the water, she faced me, I placed my hands on her shoulders, and together we shuffled into the water practicing a modified version of the fox trot. When we reached waist high water, I let go of her, splashed in on my back and began to swim over to join the others in the class who were performing a variety of water exercises.

On the weekends, we found it easier to use the Olympic-size pool that had a large area roped off for recreational use. The facility had a contraption at the edge of the pool for disabled folks like me. They'd crank me up in a pulley chair, swing me over the water, and then lower me into the pool. As my feet touched the water, I'd simply jump off the chair and begin swimming. Once in the water I was self sufficient, which meant that Terri could wander off to swim in the lap lanes. We worked this routine into our weekend schedule and stuck to it religiously throughout the year, even after I tired of the evening therapy sessions.

In the months ahead my relapse took an odd twist. My voice gradually weakened and became raspy. "Sexy," one friend said. Maybe, but I'd had to strain to be heard. We went to a vocal cord specialist who told us he suspected the neuropathy was the culprit. He tried an outpatient procedure and told me if that didn't work he could perform more involved surgery. He also said there was a good chance if I did nothing the problem would resolve on its own.

He was right, nothing more was needed. It took several months, but my voice recovered to its normal strength. I think this time at least the prednisone worked to tame any repercussions from my relapse. That was a consolation. No inkling of recovery yet, but the last thing I needed was to backslide.

The prednisone worked to my benefit in some ways, but it could also work mischief. Before the end of winter, I'd confront a new medical emergency further complicating my recovery.

Part Three: The Way Back

15 A Setback and a Strange Cure

It was early March 2001, nearly a year after my first hospitalization. I was at my office around noon, time for my first practice stroll of the day. I guided Old Mosely around my desk to my walker. For me this was a prednisone day (I was still taking 30mg of prednisone every other morning). Because prednisone is a steroid, it makes one feel stronger and decreases inflammation. The risk is that in reducing inflammation it masks the signs and symptoms of infection as well as pain. But I wasn't thinking of these risks. So in my mind, since this was a prednisone day, I should have the strength to get up from the chair into my walker on my own. Never mind that my stomach had not seemed quite right for a day or two. I had cramps and I figured maybe it was just a 48-hour bug of some sort. But I felt well enough to walk. Or so I thought. My memory of this stays with me:

I push hard on the arms of my chair in order to rise up so I might grab the side rails of the walker, first with one hand and then the other. If I succeed I have a clear path to the hallway and then it's clear sailing. No dice; try again. I close my eyes; focus, I tell myself. Sometimes I can will myself up. I'll try again. One, two, three, up. All my mental energy is focused skyward, but like a broken Jack-in-the-box, I go nowhere. Not today.

I'll phone Terri to come down from her office, just one flight up, to give me a boost. She's in the habit of bringing me a sandwich or salad for lunch every day anyhow, so it won't be an extra burden on her. But how maddening. I'm a year into this son-of-a-bitch neuropathy with no sign of gaining strength.

I motor back to my desk and dial my wife's number. Soon she appears at my door, my lunch in hand. She could see my exasperation. "My poor sweetie," she says. I motor to the front of my desk where I left my walker. Terri is small at five foot two, but her legs are strong and she's been taught how to lift me from a chair without putting out her back. She bends her knees and pulls me up. I reach for my walker and holding the side rails with each hand, I step into it. Terri gives me a hug, places my sandwich on my desk, and heads back to work.

The distance from my corner office at the end of the hall to the mailboxes near the locked entrance to the suite is, I suppose, about 50 feet. It is my routine to walk to the mailboxes, turn around and shuffle back to my office. I do this twice a day, morning and afternoon. My colleagues, hard at work in their offices, and the secretaries occupying cubicles in the hall are accustomed to my routine and pay me little mind.

Now, as I reach the mailboxes, I turn with my walker. All of a sudden my legs give way, and I collapse hard to the floor. Mai Fei, a young lawyer working with her door open, sees me go down. She remembers my ankle sprain from the day of the Christmas party last year. She dials Terri's number. "He's down," she says.

One of the secretaries rushes over. "Are you okay?" she asks. I wiggle my ankles back and forth and rub my knees. This time I seem to be fine.

"I think so," I say. Two or three hearty souls lift me up off the floor and pivot me into a chair. By now, several more colleagues—lawyers, paralegals, clerical workers—are gathered around me. I explain to the small crowd that my stomach hasn't been right the past two days. In truth, I feel ashamed of my botched effort to complete a simple walk and search for the only plausible excuse I could think of. Also, I'm embarrassed about causing such a stir in the middle of a workday. It doesn't occur to me that I could be a lot sicker than just having some 48-hour bug.

"You shouldn't be at work if you don't feel well," someone says

"Go home and rest."

I see Terri has joined the others. Her face shows concern, a tightness in her mouth. But she's gotten adept at masking her fear. She cautiously steers Old Mosely from my office, angling it so that she (or anyone else) will be able to transfer me into my wheelchair. Now, safely back in Old Mosely, she ushers me downstairs to the garage and helps transfer me into our Subaru so we can go home.

Once home, I rest, eat only broth for dinner, and take a pass on doing physical therapy. Still, neither Terri nor I entertain a thought that there is anything to be alarmed about. I go to bed early thinking the extra rest will help me get over my harmless little bug.

It was not to be. The next morning, after my usual routine of juice, coffee and newspaper time, I arose from my lift chair into my walker and headed to the bathroom. Again my knees gave way and I fell straight down. I was unhurt but getting me up would be way too difficult for just the two of us, and we knew it. Terri was adept at lifting me from a sitting position, but hauling me up from the floor was something else.

"I'll call Walter, and maybe he can find someone to help," Terri said. Walter was the building manager. He came right away, and, after assessing the situation, promptly enlisted the help of Hector, one of the all-purpose handymen (although I don't think peeling me off the ground was supposed to be one of his several purposes).

"I'll help you up," Walter said, as he placed his arm under mine, ready to lift. It quickly became obvious though, that I'd need more help than that. Even when I felt relatively good, I had no more strength than a toddler. Now I was dead weight, like a fallen tree trunk. Hector came around behind me, bent his legs and, like a champion weightlifter, raised me straight up to my feet. The two men then lugged me to the lift chair. "You better call the doctor," Walter suggested to Terri, although she had resolved to do just that without the need for prompting.

Terri left a message with Dr. Sherman's office and within minutes the doctor called back. He instructed Terri to take my temperature. I didn't feel feverish. The thermometer said otherwise. 104 degrees. Dr. Sherman then told Terri to take me to the emergency room at GW immediately. Here we go again, I thought.

Because I couldn't walk, even with assistance, Terri called for an ambulance. Mayra, our Guatemalan cleaning lady, arrived at the same time as the ambulance paramedics. Confused and startled, she watched helplessly as the paramedics lifted me into a manual wheelchair. With me in the ambulance and Terri following close behind, we headed back to familiar territory—my fifth trip to the hospital since the onset of my illness.

It didn't take long for the attendants in the emergency room to tell that I had appendicitis. X-rays further showed a perforation, making my condition all the more dangerous. We were stunned at this latest development. We had both felt certain that they would simply treat me for the flu and send me home. Apparently the prednisone had masked my condition over the last couple of days. Otherwise, I would have doubled over in pain and been whisked off to the hospital that much sooner. Instead, I went to the office with a ruptured appendix, thinking I'd just tough out a minor stomach bug. Prednisone is often thought of as a miracle drug that alleviates suffering for just about anything. Only now it seemed the villain, unless, as I'd come to suspect much later, this whole episode might actually, incomprehensibly, have been a blessing.

The hospital staff scheduled me for surgery that afternoon. I removed my wedding ring for Terri to hold while I went under the knife. We just looked at each other. We didn't have to mouth the words: *What next.*

The surgery went surprisingly well. I remember waking up in the ICU with a tube down my throat causing great discomfort, but I don't recall much else. Terri later told me that I had awakened soon after the surgery and frantically tried to pull the tubes out, causing the doctors to administer more anesthesia. But I can't recall any of that.

Fortunately, I needed only a few days in the hospital, pumped with steroids and God knows what else, to recover. I would not be going right home, however. Due to the ongoing effects of my

CIDP, coupled with the impact of surgery (the surgeon cautioned that ordinarily it takes 30 days after surgery for the body to get back to normal), the doctors prescribed a minimum of one week in the rehabilitation unit. This was the same place where I'd spent several weeks working with physical and occupational therapists almost one year earlier. I looked forward to seeing Beth, Michelle and all the gang once again. I fully expected to cry on their collective shoulders about my lack of progress to date and insist on getting better now.

Dr. Philip Marion was the head of the rehabilitation unit at GW Hospital. I had met him during my first stay there during the spring of 2000 but hadn't gotten to know him then. A tall, handsome, black man, I now found him affable, forthright and easy to talk to. He stopped by my room as soon as I was admitted to rehab.

"My greatest concern for you is respiratory," he said. "What has so far been your saving grace is your physical fitness. Patients in your condition often need a ventilator."

Dr. Marion was also an avid runner. We chatted about each other's running prowess. He was impressed that before my illness I had been a seven-minute miler. Like me, he lived in Cleveland Park and we discussed our favorite running routes. He explained that I'd be expected to spend three hours each day in physical and occupational therapy, broken into 45-minute sessions. I joked that the doctors had me on so many steroids that I'd have a hard time qualifying for the Olympics.

Before he left, he repeated that my physical conditioning, particularly my running routine, probably had spared me from having to be placed on a ventilator during my first stay in the hospital. I told him that I was eager to get back to my normal routine, so that my recovery could begin at long last.

I didn't mention that I'd been feeling discouraged that a year or more had passed since my early signs of illness, and that real progress—progress beyond my modest gains through physical therapy—was nonexistent. I didn't want to appear to be a whiner. But, Dr. Richardson's words continued to play on my mind like an old, tired show tune. If I couldn't regain strength in eighteen months, if the peripheral nerves didn't re-connect with the muscles by then, my muscles would almost assuredly start to waste and I'd never get better. This thought had been haunting me day and night for nearly a year. Now, with the added setback of the surgery, I feared that the eighteen-month deadline was slipping beyond my grasp.

I wound up spending two weeks in rehab. I worked hard enough; Beth even told me that my work ethic made it seem as if I was preparing for the Olympics. To my great disappointment, however, I was unable to perform, even at the modest level that Billie had had me at before the appendectomy disrupted my home routine.

In physical therapy sessions with Beth, I'd do a regimen of leg exercises in the morning. My hamstrings proved to be my weakest muscles. I would lay on my stomach attempting to raise my legs, first my right, then my left, but they wouldn't budge. My quads performed a little better, but not much. I suffered from what is commonly called "foot drop" which comes from weak dorsiflexion. When Terri came in the evenings, she would stand at the bottom of my bed flexing my feet up and down, which, we were told, would prevent a contraction if done regularly. I didn't suffer from much pain, but I still experienced occasional buzzing in my feet, somewhat like mini electric shocks. This feeling was annoying but not so painful. I took a drug called Neurontin to ease this sensation but that did me little good.

In the afternoon, Beth had me sit in a small booth, a contraption designed to determine at what height I could rise from a sitting position. She would start with the seat lowered and crank it up a little at a time until it was high enough for me to simply pop up. Beth puzzled as to why I couldn't get up more easily because she said my gluts were relatively strong.

Beth said that I was too weak for walking to be a focus of my therapy at this time; however, at my insistence, she incorporated walking, with the use of my walker and safety belt, as part of the afternoon routine.

She repeated what she'd told me a year earlier. "No one would be walking with leg muscles so weak. You compensate for your legs by leaning too hard on the walker with your arms. I worry about your falling."

But I told her that I'd been walking every day at home, as well as at the office, back and forth, along the corridors outside my apartment. Even if just as a boost to my morale, I wanted to keep it up. One time, toward the end of a tiring session I did fall, spraining my ankle slightly. In spite of my determination, Beth suspended further walking exercises after that incident.

The occupational therapy exercises were less stressful this time around. Michelle timed me while I placed pegs in holes on a small board. I had very little movement in my fingers and my wrists were still very weak, so I worked on a variety of exercises meant to provide greater dexterity. I also lifted five-pound dumbbells, pretending I was Arnold Schwarzenegger.

Nearing the end of my time in rehab I showed no improvement in strength whatsoever. But it was now just one month since my surgery. The surgeon had cautioned that it would take that long for my metabolism to get back to normal, so I remained hopeful despite the lack of progress. Beth gave me leg braces, which locked my knees, whenever it was necessary for me to walk, even if just to the bathroom. She further instructed Terri to crawl on all fours behind me, a hand on each leg, whenever I walked, at least until we could be confident that I could go short distances on my own. What an arduous routine, we both thought.

I told Jane about all of this, about the cumbersome routine we'd have to undergo at home, when she came to visit that afternoon. Jane said that she and other friends of ours had talked about the need to give Terri a break from caring for me. "Michael, we're not sure you realize the pressure on Terri day in and day out. There's a danger that she'll burn out. I'm speaking to you as a friend. As much as Terri cares for you, you need to think about hiring a nurse's aide, at least on weekends. Terri needs her own time or she'll exhaust herself physically and emotionally and you don't want that."

I was taken aback by the forcefulness of Jane's suggestion and the possibility that, indeed, I'd been selfish in not thinking about giving Terri more free time. None of this had dawned on me. I suddenly felt like a heartless fool. I brought it up with Terri that evening as soon as she walked in the door, but she immediately rejected the idea of hiring a companion for me.

"Do we really want some stranger in a white uniform showing up every Saturday?

"Really, we'll make out just fine. You've never held me back from running or taking a bike ride, and if I wanted to disappear for a day to go hiking or something like that, I know you'd be okay with it. But honestly, that's not at the top of my list. Remember, I said we're in this together—and I meant that. Let's keep it just us, okay?"

In truth, Terri was apprehensive about whether she was capable of handling me in my severely debilitated state, losing sleep as the day for my discharge drew closer. She didn't let on about her worries until much later, but she also felt pangs of guilt that she could still enjoy a brisk morning run, when I could barely lift myself out of bed. She knew, intellectually, that she needed that time to herself, and she'd always return feeling refreshed and renewed and braced for any surprises I might have in store for her. Yet under her bravado, she worried deep down what life would be like if I could never walk again.

If only, like reading a good mystery novel, I could page forward to see what would happen, how this would all turn out in the end, but that was not an option. Instead I thought back, as I had time and again, on what is known about my condition, on all the treatments that were tried and failed, and where I stood now.

The medical evidence suggests without certainty that CIDP is caused by the body's immune system. It is equally true that we might as well be living in the dark ages for all that medical science knows about our immune systems. The components of our immune systems—anti-bodies, certain plasma proteins, and white blood cells—normally act to fend off viruses and infections. That's their job. However, in some disorders, such as Guillain-Barre Syndrome and CIDP, the immune system, although well meaning, screws up and reacts against parts of our bodies, causing disease. It is thought that this happens when a particular virus or infection mimics certain parts of our body, thereby instigating an attack.

Although the cause of CIDP is not well understood, what is known is that up to eighty percent of CIDP patients respond to one or more treatments that impact the immune system in some way. *By now, I had tried all of these treatments. None had worked.*

At first, the neurologists at GW had put me on prednisone, the miracle steroid that they thought would improve strength and reduce inflammation. Simultaneously, they arranged for intravenous immunoglobulin (IVIgG) therapy once a month. This treatment, a sterile solution of concentrated highly purified antibodies taken from thousands of healthy people, is given through a vein in the forearm either in an out-patient facility or by an infusion service at home. The idea, I suppose, is to trick the immune system into thinking it won the battle allowing its soldiers to go home. Improvement can be expected in a matter of days and may last from three to six weeks. However, I saw no improvement with this regimen; I only got worse to the point of not being able to walk. That's when I embarked upon my first hospitalization in April 2000. My illness was winning.

In the hospital they kept me on prednisone and implemented a plasma exchange procedure known as plasmapheresis, whereby plasma is removed from the blood and replaced with a new fluid. This procedure, which is repeated every other day over the course of one week, is done through a catheter that is inserted into a large vein under the collarbone or thereabouts. Plasmapheresis is safe and causes rapid improvement in many patients. I was not among them, however. CIDP had bested three known treatments so far.

The final, last-gasp, treatment I received was a once a month, six-month course of Cytoxan, a chemotherapy given primarily to cancer patients. The intent here was to suppress my immune system enough to halt its attack on my peripheral nerves. By March 2001, six months had come and gone and I wasn't seeing progress. And I was out of options, or so I thought. CIDP 4, me 0.

What I couldn't have known, or even suspected, was that this whole episode involving my appendix might actually be a blessing. As my internist, Dr. Sherman would later—much later—theorize, my ruptured appendix required the full attention of my immune system in order to properly heal following surgery. Accordingly, like soldiers who had mistakenly engaged in friendly fire and were subsequently re-directed to the battle front, my anti-bodies and their minions were directed away from their attack on my peripheral nerves toward fighting off a genuine foe—the infection that might arise from my ruptured appendix. In other words, after successfully fending off infection from the appendectomy, my immune system abandoned its attack on my body, and in so doing, allowed the slow process of recovery of my damaged peripheral nerves to begin in earnest. Such was Dr. Sherman's theory.

A rather strange cure, indeed, and not one I could anticipate during these last few days in the hospital or anytime soon.

16 March Madness at the Hospital

Despite continued uncertainty about my future, my mental state was somewhat different than it had been during my first hospital stay in April 2000. Then I'd been frightened at my new predicament, uncertain whether I could cope day-to-day, challenged by simple tasks at home like taking a shower or making my lunch. I was also unwilling to contemplate that my condition could be anything other than temporary, two months maybe, at worst, four months. I was alarmed to hear that I had, at most, 18 months to recover use of my muscles. "Muscles are forgiving," Dr. Richardson, my neurologist, had said, "but only up to a point. After 18 months, your muscles won't recognize your nerves and wasting will occur." The message kept replaying in my head: however I found myself after 18 months would be my permanent state of being.

Now, nearly a year had passed and here I was again, in the hospital for weeks on end, still plagued by uncertainty. If I'd known a year ago that I'd have no hint of recovery by this time, I'd most likely have fallen into despair. But by now, Terri and I had established a workable routine at home. With the help of Old Mosely, I was back at work, leading big cases just as before, albeit without the travel. As senior counsel, I could delegate travel for such things as depositions or meeting with expert witnesses to other lawyers assigned to my trial team. Also, with Old Mosely, I could ride the metro alone so long as the elevators were working.

Please, oh please, let the elevator at Metro Center be working. And I still had the help of Billie, my physical therapist, two evenings a week, while faithfully lifting weights and walking the corridors outside my apartment with my walker on other days. Friends and work colleagues, as well as my doctors and therapists, were all applauding me for coping and striving to get better while continuing with work, play, and all of the stuff of life. "So many people in your situation would crumble," one friend told me.

The weird thing is that all my life I'd gotten so exasperated when little things didn't go my way. If my vacation flight was delayed or I couldn't find my keys when in a hurry, torrents of curses would flow from my lips like storm water from a roof. I would have thought that I'd be the last person on earth to endure something this big in a cool and collected way. Not that I was cool and collected—I was nervous and worried as hell—but I suppose I maintained a certain outward composure.

But also, I had changed in some way. I wasn't as snappish, Terri observed. I came to understand that if little things go wrong they can be fixed. Now that I had a real fight on my hands, it no longer made sense to sweat the small stuff. Some people mellow with age. I suppose I'd mellowed with disease. Still, the medical set backs over the past year and uncertainty of what was to come made me hungrier than ever for a semblance of normality and lighthearted diversion. Maybe even a bit of mischief.

One of the pluses of spending March in rehab was being able to watch many of the first and second round games of the men's NCAA basketball tournament. I was addicted to "March Madness"; it was my one and only vice in the category of vicarious sports obsession. The 32 games played in the first round occurred in mid-March, and one-half of those games were televised during the day. That made it difficult to tune in while working a day job, but for this short spell I was on leave from my day job.

The rooms in rehab were private, one-person rooms, so working around my therapy schedule, I tuned into those games that I cared about. Judy, an ex-colleague and good friend who was a sports nut of the first order, phoned me to ask if she could stop by on Sunday for a visit. This meant that we'd watch some of the second round games. As there were no therapy sessions held on Sundays, I told her I'd be free all afternoon and into the evening. I primarily rooted for Maryland and the other ACC teams. I noticed that North Carolina would be on at 5 p.m. on Sunday, which would allow Terri, Judy and me time to enjoy a sports-free visit before the game. Terri committed to picking up a carryout dinner for all of us for later, while Judy and I were focused on the game.

Judy and I had worked together in the Torts Branch for many years. She left sometime in the mid-90's to become first a magistrate and later a judge with the D.C. Superior Court. A robust, tall, muscular woman, Judy is a larger than life personality whose presence lights up a room. She enjoys just about every aspect of life—not just sports—to the fullest (with the possible exception of cooking). Her booming laughter is infectious. She's never afraid to express an opinion on any topic, but she'll always listen intently to the views of others. She's simply great fun to be with. Judy is also one of the most traveled people I know, having explored everywhere from Mongolia to the Amazon. I took a walking trip with her husband Vince and son Joel in Sicily, about a year before I met Terri. I'll always cherish the memories of that trip, meandering through fields thick with gorse, visiting cobbled hill towns, and enjoying the sumptuous lunchtime picnics. Sports might have been Judy's favorite thing of all, however, and so, I looked forward to her upcoming visit to watch the Carolina game.

When Judy arrived on Sunday, she scoped my quarters and soon surmised that, while the room seemed comfortable enough for a hospital setting, the TV was awfully small and it might be more fun to go for a walk and seek out a cozy bar where we could watch the game over beers and burgers. I knew that just a couple of blocks east of the hospital, on the edge of the GW University campus, there was a small indoor shopping mall which had deli restaurants and a bar or two. So Judy's suggestion was feasible, assuming we could get permission from Pat, the charge nurse on duty on Sundays. Hospital rules prohibited patients from wandering off the hospital grounds, but Terri sweet-talked Pat into allowing us to bend the rules, just a wee bit, by assuring her that we'd go for a short walk, get a Starbucks coffee and come right back.

"That's okay," Pat said, "but try to be back in 15 minutes. Remember, I am responsible for him."

"Oh, we will," Terri said. I'm sure that Terri experienced a momentary pang of guilt for this fib. I know that I did. We both liked Pat. She was pleasant, supportive, and happy to do us small favors, such as making me a cup of coffee from the tin of Café Francais that Terri brought in for me. But now we were set on this outing, and we needed to tell a white lie in order to make a smooth getaway.

So out we went on this spring-like day in mid-March. I was dressed in pajama bottoms and a t-shirt. In light of the weather, I felt no need to change for the occasion. I also had on my hospital identification band that had been fastened on my wrist the day of my surgery. At least I wasn't wearing one of the ubiquitous blue and white hospital gowns that open in the back. I'd given up that attire some time before, after an elderly roommate had mooned me while bending over the clothes bureau.

We headed down I Street toward the shops on Pennsylvania Avenue. As Terri rolled my wheelchair along, I felt giddy with freedom. I was an escapee from GW Hospital. I felt like I had just robbed a bank. I looked back imagining nurses and attendants in hot pursuit, but there were only Sunday strollers and GW students. We entered the shops and searched for a deli or bar with a TV. One lunch spot was closed and a small bar would not open for two hours. But Judy noticed that Kinkead's, an upscale restaurant, was open for business.

"I can't go in there," I protested. "Not dressed like this."

"Come on," Judy said. "It's early. No one's there yet. We can sit in the bar and watch the game." The maitre d' graciously sat us at a table in the bar area and turned on the game for us. North Carolina was losing badly with no sign of gaining momentum. We soon turned our attention away from the game. We ordered a bottle of merlot and appetizers. We drank the wine, chatted and laughed and ordered more wine. We were having a good time and one thing led to another. We each ordered an entree. I ordered duck. Judy got the steak. Kinkead's was best known for its seafood and fish. Terri ordered scallops. Before long, more and more people streamed in for dinner.

"I better give Pat a call," Terri said suddenly. "It's been a helluva lot longer than 15 minutes."

"Go ahead," I said. "Pat's cool; she won't mind our being a little late. Call her." Terri left the table to phone Pat.

When she returned, Terri recounted the awkward conversation she'd just had with Pat. "You are WHERE? You get him back here this instant. I am responsible for him," Pat had said.

"I told her we just ordered our dinner," Terri said.

"Well get him back as soon as you finish," Pat had said, again explaining that she was solely responsible for me and would pay a big price if anything happened.

That difficult mission accomplished, we resumed our dinner. I occasionally looked around the restaurant to see if anyone was noticing my less than formal attire. My self-consciousness was misplaced. We drank, we ate, and we ordered dessert. Judy's favorite, apple tarte tatin, was on the menu. It would take an extra 30 minutes to prepare.

"I had the most exceptional tarte Tatin once on a ski trip in northern Italy," Judy said. "I've tried to recreate that experience ever since but haven't found anything like it. I simply MUST have the tarte Tatin. Do you mind the extra wait? I'll take full responsibility. Blame it on me."

"I guess a few extra minutes won't matter," Terri said. Judy went on to explain in detail why she'd liked the tarte Tatin in Italy so much. I leaned over to Terri.

"I'm getting a little nervous about being out so long," I whispered. "Pat was very plain about our need to get back soon. She's responsible for me."

"But Judy really wants it. I don't know what else to do. Let her order it, and we'll hurry straight back."

After dinner we checked the time. I'd been AWOL for about three hours. We said good-bye to Judy who wished us good luck in avoiding a dressing down upon our return. Terri and I walked the four blocks back to the hospital, voicing the hope that Pat would be away from her station when we exited the elevator on the fifth floor, so that we could slink back into my room unnoticed. We were two little kids returning home, our pockets full of candy, conspiring to avoid Mama by sneaking through the back door.

"I want to see you in your room right now," Pat snarled as soon as the elevator doors opened. We headed straight to my room with Pat close behind. She strode in and closed the door behind her. When she saw our sorrowful faces, she quickly softened and, almost apologetically, explained the nature of her responsibility. She knew I was to be discharged in a few days.

"I don't want to be a hard ass, but you must know that the hospital could be liable for any mishap while you're a patient," Pat explained again. "I'd be held responsible by the hospital if anything happened to you."

"We're really very sorry, Pat," Terri said, ever the diplomat. "One thing led to another. We never ever intended to stay away this long. It won't happen again, we promise."

"Does this mean I'll get a dishonorable discharge?" I asked, putting on my saddest puppy-dog face.

Pat laughed. Everything was okay again. In two or three days I was discharged. Honorably, I think.

Within one or two days after returning home, I felt strong enough to walk without the knee-locking braces that Beth had prescribed. I resumed physical therapy with Billie, as well as my daily walks, and suffered no mishaps. I seemed to be just about as strong as before the appendectomy. The doctor's prognosis concerning a 30-day recovery was on the money. Whether I'd continue to improve any further remained to be seen. Two thirds of my 18-month allotted recovery time had already passed. Six months left.

17 Sign of the Times

We flew up to Boston the second weekend in September 2001 to help Jessica settle in for her second (and final) year at Lesley College. She'd done well in her classes her first year and was leaning toward a career in elderly care, perhaps helping to run a recreational program for assisted living residents. She'd job shadow in that field this coming year before making up her mind. We had dinner with Jessica and a few of her friends Saturday evening and flew back to D.C. on Sunday.

The next morning, we prepared to go to work like any other weekday. We arose around 6 a.m. I transferred from the bed to Old Mosely and rolled to the lift chair in the living room. Terri brought in the paper and brought me orange juice and coffee. We turned on the radio, tuning in to WGMS, the classical music station. Soothing music to wake up by. I browsed through the paper, first the front section and then the sports. Terri looked through the Style section and skimmed the front section when I had finished. There wasn't much in the news then as I recall. Chandra Levy was still missing and Connie Chung was being scolded for her overly aggressive interview of Gary Condit, the congressman suspected of involvement in Chandra's disappearance.

When newspaper time was over, I transferred from Old Mosely to the recumbent bike. Terri tied my feet to the pedals as otherwise they had a habit of slipping out. Then she went for a run in nearby Rock Creek Park. I would pedal hard on the bike until she got back. Again, a typical work week morning.

At some point WGMS interrupted the music with a news bulletin reporting that a small aircraft had hit the World Trade Center. I was puzzled but thought little of it. When Terri returned from her run, we took turns showering. After getting dressed for work, we turned on CNN to learn that the President was about to speak. Apparently, a commercial airliner, not a small plane, had hit the second building of the World Trade Center. By now, it was clear that this incident in New York was related to terrorism. We stayed to hear what President Bush had to say. No harm, we supposed, with a short delay in getting to work. Still, the seriousness of the situation hadn't fully dawned on us. There seemed no reason not to get on with the day.

We got the car out of the garage, loaded Old Mosely into the hatch, and drove east along Park Road to Thirteenth Street, as usual, and then south on Thirteenth to our downtown office. As we were driving, the news broke that a third plane had hit the Pentagon. In heading south toward downtown on any number of north-south streets past Meridian Hill, the streets start to slope downward yielding views that take in a wide swath of the downtown area, including the Washington Monument, the Jefferson Memorial, and, further out to the northern suburbs of Virginia. At this point, we could see what we figured had to be smoke rising from the Pentagon.

In hindsight, I wish we'd stopped, turned around and headed home. But we didn't, we held tight to the path taking us to a typical workday. As we entered the lobby of our office building from The Shops (an indoor mall) on F Street, people were streaming out. I saw our friend Gay among the throng. "What's going on?" I asked.

"We've all been told to leave. You guys better turn around and go home."

"I've just got to go up to my office for a quick second," Terri said. "Michael, wait here, I'll be right down."

I parked Old Mosely against a wall, out of the way of the crowd and waited. The concierge of the building, an affable woman who I greeted every morning, came out from behind her desk and over to me. She had tears in her eyes. "You better be off, I just got word that they hit the Capitol and the White House." Rumors were rampant. She seemed about to lose it.

"I'm just waiting for my wife. She'll be right down."

"Alright then."

Terri returned with her book bag in tow after about ten minutes. "I was watching the TV in the conference room with Mike and Chris. One of the twin trade tower buildings just collapsed. We better get the hell outta here."

We headed straight back to the garage, got the car and drove out the gate and into one of the most chaotic scenes in memory:

There's no use in trying to turn left, so Terri turns right. We can circle the block and turn north on Fourteenth Street. Several colleagues of mine are mulling outside the Marriott across from Freedom Plaza. I stick my head out of the car window and wave to them. "We're going to hole up in a café and wait out the traffic," one of them calls out to us.

"You have a good thought there," I holler back. "Too late for us to join you. Maybe, if we're lucky, we'll make it home by nightfall."

It takes us over a half hour to poke over to Fourteenth Street. Traffic is barely moving there. "Let's head east," I say. "Maybe other streets will be less jam packed."

We try several other northbound streets in the hopes of breaking away from the battling throngs. All the streets heading north are clogged. "Let's try Sixth Street," Terri says without much conviction.

In about two hours we make it out of the downtown area. After a while, the congestion starts to ease. It occurs to us that we are all sitting ducks should the terrorists decide to strike at downtown. "Please let's not see a plane overhead," I implore. Why in god's name did the powers that be decide that everyone who'd gone to work should turn right around in unison? Don't they have the least bit of horse sense?"

"They are clueless," Terri says. "Clueless. Just plain clueless. How can this be happening?"

I'm so relieved when at last we pull into the garage of our condo building.

We made it home in a little over three hours, not as bad as it could have been. We turned on CNN. Mayor Giuliani was shown repeating that there had to have been an enormous loss of life with the collapse of the buildings. No mention, thank goodness, of attacks on the Capitol or the White House. Just false rumors. But the enormity of the day's events was starting to sink in.

We tried calling Jessica's cell phone but the circuits were busy. She eventually reached us. She seemed to be doing fine. "Has Kate contacted her mother yet?" Terri asked. Kate was Jessica's roommate. Her mother, Barbara, worked at the Pentagon.

"No, not yet. Kate's really worried." We tried calling Barbara at her home and left a message. Later she called back. Fortunately, she'd been on assignment elsewhere that morning, but she knew several folks who'd been in harm's way, maybe even killed, and she was shaken. By now, however, she'd spoken to her daughter. She thanked us for calling. After hanging up, we took a deep breath.

We sat transfixed before the TV in the days that followed. We were moved to tears by the people holding up signs seeking news, any news, of their missing loved ones. All of a sudden the nation was shocked, and its citizens ever more vulnerable. Nothing like this had occurred in recent history. I wasn't around for Pearl Harbor. JFK's assassination was the one tragic event that was at all comparable to 9/11 in my memory. I'd been 16 then.

As for me, I came to realize that everything is relative. I might have this odd illness that came upon me out of the blue, but at least I was alive. In the context of the events of 9/11, I felt lucky. After all, we'd just flown back from Boston the day before. What if we'd delayed our return trip one day? One of the planes that crashed had taken off from Boston.

But in the days and weeks ahead I began to feel personally vulnerable. Or, perhaps, more to the point, I began to obsess about all the bad things that could happen. Whenever Terri went out, to go shopping or marketing, or to girl's night with her friends, or just for a jog in the park, I'd worry that she might not make it back. What would I do then? I'd be lost without her. At the office I was assigned a person to stick with me during fire drills. I couldn't take Old Mosely down the stairs so my monitor would assure I got safely down on the elevator and back up again after the all clear signal was given. But at home Terri was my whole world. I depended on her to get me through each day: help me shower, help me dress, drive to work. Without her I couldn't function. *If the terrorists were to get one of us, let it be me.* Every time she went out, for whatever reason, I breathed a sigh of relief when she came back, the sound of her keys jingling in the lock.

We were lucky compared to the victims of that day but vulnerable. Oh so vulnerable.

18 Where Will We Call Home?

In October, Terri and I took a trip to San Diego to explore the possibility of moving there. By now, a full eighteen months had elapsed since my initial hospitalization back in April 2000. It was time to take stock. Maybe it would be good to live some place where the weather was agreeable year round.

In recent weeks my arms were gaining strength, so I had reason to be hopeful. The doctors had been both too optimistic and too pessimistic. At first, they'd thought my diagnosis was all good news. They'd put too much stock in treatments they thought would yield a quick recovery. But when those treatments failed to show results, they fixated on the 18-month scenario. Were they back-peddling now? During a recent visit, Dr. Richardson had been pleased to chart my progress. "There's no reason you shouldn't continue to improve," he'd said. I saw no purpose in reminding him that my 18-month deadline for recovery was about to expire.

Of course, I still couldn't fend for myself. I couldn't yet get up out of my wheelchair on my own, and I dreaded being immobile during the cold winters. My hands and feet always felt like ice cubes after going outdoors for only a few minutes. Why not relocate to a warmer climate with a more relaxed lifestyle?

So we pondered the feasibility of such a move. I'd soon be eligible for retirement, which would carry with it a healthy pension due to 30 years of government service. We were confident that

Terri could easily find immigration law work in southern California. Also, Terri's cousins, Steve and Odile, lived just north of San Diego. I hadn't gotten to know them yet, but for Terri's sake, they'd provide a family connection.

Also, Jessica would be completing her two-year vocational program in Boston in less than a year. When the time came for her to return home from school for good, we knew that she and her long-term beau, Daniel, would almost certainly be around much of the time. We were still in our Connecticut Avenue apartment. The place was way too small for us all. We'd put off buying a house because of my illness, but clearly we could delay no longer.

While neither Terri nor I had been to San Diego, we'd heard about its idyllic Mediterranean climate and knew from our readings that it was a lovely city surrounded by waters and mountains. Also, of particular importance to us both, we understood it to be a wheelchair friendly place. So a west coast sojourn seemed like an apt and timely adventure. We planned a two-week trip for late October.

We weren't without misgivings about the prospect of moving west. Indeed, as I reflect on this period of my illness, I sometimes wonder: *What could I have been thinking*? My illness was being monitored by my doctors who were familiar with my medical needs and history. Finding new specialists would be a daunting task. Also, I didn't want to abandon Jessica who would just be starting out in the work force. Would she move out west with us or stay behind with Daniel? If the latter, surely she'd still need the safety net that only we could provide. Terri too felt uncertain about having to care for me without the support of family and friends.

"I don't know, Michael. All of our friends, everyone who has been helping us through this crisis, they're all here. What'll you do, who will you talk to when I'm at work? I'd worry about you. I can't do it all myself."

"Don't jump the gun. We're not moving yet. Let's explore the possibility and enjoy the trip one way or another. Let's just keep an open mind."

But Terri had a point. Her cousins, by themselves, could hardly be expected to provide the kind of support system we'd be leaving behind. She was also anxious and uncertain about the prospect of starting a new job on top of the move and caring for me. Our friends at home cautioned us about the perils of uprooting ourselves too hastily. Nevertheless, an exploratory adventure couldn't hurt.

So, in October, we flew across the country. We had booked a hotel on Mission Bay just two blocks from the ocean. In the wake of 9-11, very few people were traveling. We were told we could probably stay anywhere, including the renowned Coronado Beach Hotel, for half price. We were happy with the place we'd chosen. We had also reserved a motorized scooter for me. These are generally faster than chairs, and if I liked it enough I might buy one when we got back home. The fellow who rented the scooter to us delivered it to our hotel and gave me a lesson in driving it. Then he showed Terri how to break it down so she could fit it into the trunk of our rental car. The scooter broke down into three parts, which turned out to be less complicated than disassembling Old Mosely. Lifting these hefty parts up and into the trunk was another matter. But somehow, my petite wife, with some heaving, shoving and cursing, managed it.

After settling in, we explored our surroundings. The rear of the hotel opened out to Mission Bay and the hotel's own little complex of docks. Several small boats were secured with lines to the piers jutting out from the docks. A pedestrian path separated the hotel from the docks and the path appeared to encircle the bay, at least as far as we could see. I was immediately envious of Terri, who could take full advantage of this venue for her early morning runs. I gazed with envy also upon the mid-afternoon bicyclers and joggers as they whizzed by enjoying the scenery as well as the mental high that I knew they were feeling from the release of pent-up energy. I could ride my scooter along the path while Terri went for a jog, but I'd sorely miss the pleasure of running or biking against this colorful landscape at dawn's break. With all the waterways and ocean beaches, San Diego is a runner's paradise.

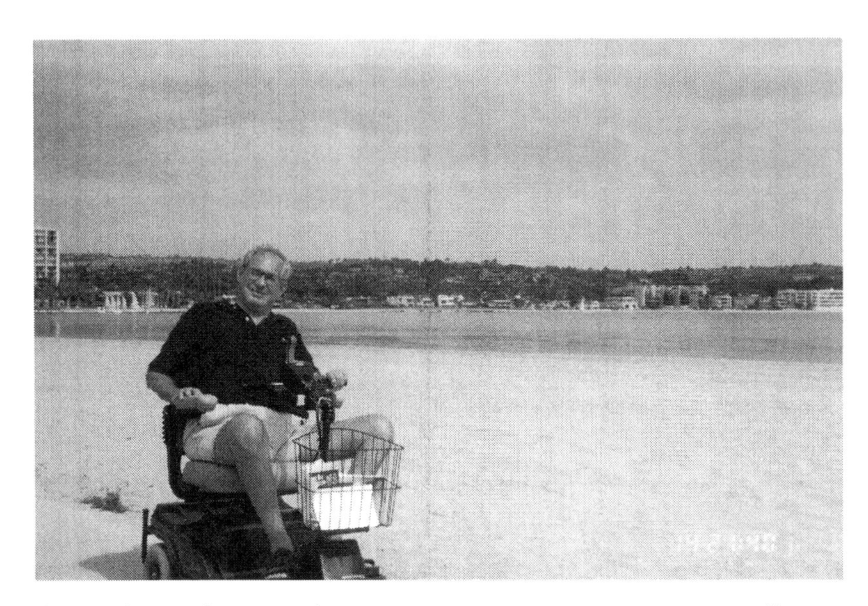

The author in his rental scooter, Mission Bay, San Diego, Fall 2001

Even though we were on holiday, we took seriously the notion that we might decide to move to San Diego within a year or two. We contacted a real estate agent who insisted on taking us around to neighborhoods he thought we should see. If we moved here we'd want to at least be within a short walk of the ocean. La Jolla proved too hilly for me in my chair and too pricey. Coronado Beach was flat and lovely, resembling parts of the French Riviera, but also unaffordable. Pacific Beach was within our range and had a scenic and accessible oceanfront. Perfect for rolling in my chair or scooter or for walking. This was important because, like a preacher who believes in the coming of the messiah, I maintained absolute faith in my ability to walk again.

Our agent was so patient with us, helping Terri lift and assemble the scooter and then disassemble it each time we stopped to look at a house. We felt guilty for taking his time and energy, but he was insistent. "Those are the risks we take in the trade," he explained, in response to our uncertainty as to when or whether we planned to move. Later, he faxed information to our hotel so that we could explore more neighborhoods on our own in the coming days. We felt as if he'd given us the full tour. And I was getting more and more excited about the prospect of moving to this paradise by the sea.

During the second week of our stay, Terri interviewed with the U.S. Attorney's office that was looking to hire more lawyers with immigration experience. We were confident the job was hers if we decided to pursue the move west. However, I could tell that Terri remained less excited and more stressed than I about the actuality of moving across country, while simultaneously changing jobs and caring for me. Not to mention her worries about how I might handle such a change.

Our trip wasn't all business, though. We toured all around the city that might become our new home. We visited Balboa Park, spent a morning observing the rhinos and bears at the vaunted San Diego Zoo, and gazed with awe at the hang gliders along the cliffs just north of the city. San Diego is a city of diverse neighborhoods, and we explored several of these, strolling along the coast at La Jolla, drinking cosmopolitans by the sea at Coronado Beach, and meandering along the streets of the quaint bricked gaslight district in the downtown area. We found San Diego to be just as handicap accessible as we had expected. There was nowhere that I couldn't go, either by elevator, ramp, or lift. In contrast to the towns and villages of New England, where so many of the buildings are old and rickety (having been built ages ago when disabled folks apparently never ventured outside), San Diego's walkways and sidewalks spread wide, offering cut curbs at every corner, and sometimes, in between. The city even offered for rent wheelchairs that could maneuver on sand and wade into the ocean.

One evening we dined with Terri's cousins and their two small boys at their home in Del Mar, just north of the city limits. Before dinner they showed us around the oceanfront closest to where they lived. We strolled through the lovely lush green park that follows the coast. Palm trees and lavender bougainvillea lined the path. The smaller boy was in a stroller, so I had company rolling along the coastal path. After our walk, they took us by car to view their favorite haunts. Del Mar is a cozy village with a variety of cafes, shops and restaurants. We'd have to consider looking there

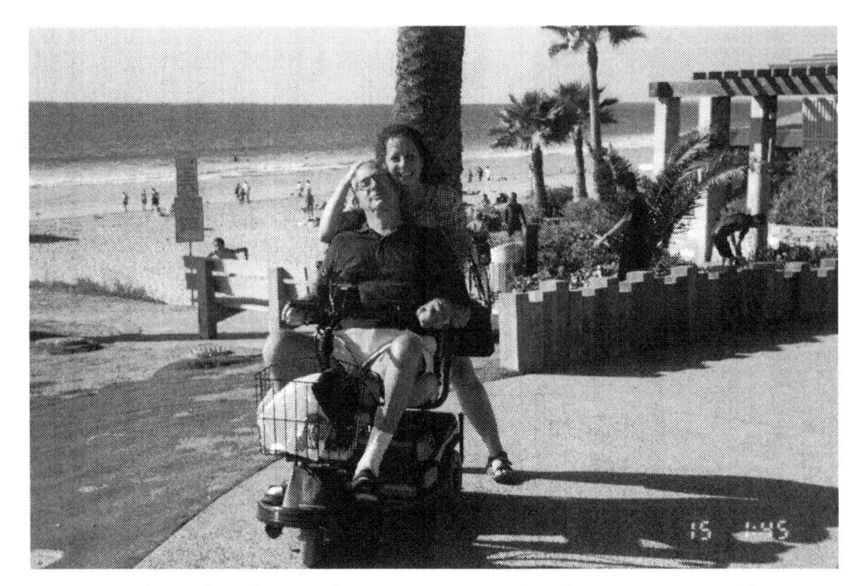

Terri and Michael in Del Mar, just north of San Diego, Fall 2001

when and if we actually made the move.

As we pulled into the driveway of their house, Steve and Odile seemed a bit taken aback by the arduous process of getting me in and out of the car. "Terri, this is quite a rigmarole you two have to go through," Steve said, as he lifted the several parts to the scooter out of the trunk.

"Yes, but we're used to it by now," Terri said. Steve lugged the parts up the steps and into the foyer. Then he watched as Terri reassembled the scooter. That done, they lifted me out of the car and helped me into the house. I stayed downstairs chatting with Steve, as Odile gave Terri the full tour.

Steve and Odile were gracious hosts and a charming couple. They'd surely provide a family connection when the time came. Even if we didn't move to San Diego, I vowed to come back and visit some day when I could walk again. "Next time you come here to visit, Michael, you'll be walking in right over this threshold," Odile said, as she escorted us out the front door and to our car.

One day during the second week of our holiday, we took their advice and set out for the historic village of Julian, a mountain retreat one hour east of San Diego. A gold mining town founded soon after the Civil War, Julian is best known today for its apples and apple pies. It is not, though, as handicap accessible as San Diego, as we found out the hard way:

We park on one of the town's quiet side streets, assemble the scooter, and set out to explore the town. The sidewalks have cut curbs, allowing my scooter to traverse them easily enough, but the streets have annoying speed bumps that pose a challenge for the likes of me. Julian is a western town that was developed in the nineteenth century, so many of the stores have wooden steps that prevent me from going inside. Nonetheless, we peek into some of the specialty shops lining the main street, and stop to sample apple pie that any number of cafes claim to be the best in town.

"You can't get the scooter inside here, but why don't you claim one of the outdoor tables. I'll go on in and get us some pie and iced coffee," Terri says.

I pull the scooter up to one of the picnic tables and wait, swatting away yellow jackets, while Terri goes inside the café to order the pie. After our respite, we roam the streets some more, but soon decide we've seen all there is to see in Julian. We resolve to head back to San Diego in time for a siesta or a stroll along the bay. Because our rental car is parked in the middle of a block off the main drag where there is no cut curb, I decide it's best for me to roll along the side of the street to the car rather than on the sidewalk. As I turn down the street, I look back. Terri is having trouble keeping up with my speedy scooter and is lagging behind by half a block. I make a game effort to tackle the one imposing speed bump that separates me from our car. Shit! My scooter is stuck at the peak of the bump. Try as I might, there is no coaxing it over the top. I back it off the bump and turn it around, driving it far enough away to get a running start. Now I'll show my stuff. I gun the motor pretending I'm a NASCAR driver. This time the scooter doesn't get stuck on the bump. Instead, it does a spiral turn in midair before landing on its side and dumping me head first onto the pavement. Horrified, my wife signals for help and a group of people come running. First, they check if I'm okay. "I think so," I say. Then they help me into the car.

Luckily, neither I nor the scooter need emergency medical attention. When Terri sees that I'm okay her fear turns to annoyance. "That was a moronic thing to do, Michael. Next time wait for me."

As it turns out, except for a temporary headache suffered during part of the return trip, I'm largely unscathed.

I do not blame the town of Julian for my mishap, only my stubborn nature. Nevertheless, I couldn't help but think that somebody up there was seeking revenge on my behalf when, sometime during the following summer, as I was watching CNN, it was reported that Julian was in imminent danger of being consumed by a wildfire. The town was ultimately spared, but many homes in the surrounding countryside were destroyed and the fire took nearly a month to be contained.

In the end, we didn't move to San Diego. Not that such a move wasn't tempting—the dry, moderate climate appealed to me, and a city surrounded by water and more distant mountains held the promise of adventure and a new life enhanced by what I fully expected to be my inevitable recovery. At the end of the day, however, we believed it unwise to simply up and leave behind my daughter, our entrenched friendships, and the care of my doctors.

During the spring of 2002, we realized that the moment was nearing when Jessica would be returning home from school and spending most of her time with Daniel at our place. Our two-bedroom condo suddenly seemed tiny. We'd come to accept that San Diego was not in our future, so we began to search for a house in the D.C. area. Hopefully, we could find something that would be reasonably accessible for Old Mosely and me.

We hired a real estate agent and reserved weekends in March and April for the hunt. We scratched colonials and townhouses off the agenda right away (too vertical). It also became painfully clear that there are very few houses out there that are strictly one level. Just about every home has some stairs to negotiate. We knew that we'd need to compromise by outfitting our new home with ramps, and perhaps, a lift or elevator to allow Old Mosely free range. But we wanted a horizontal house, and toward that end, we focused primarily on ramblers and split-levels.

Danny, our real estate agent, arranged to show us a house near White Oak. Jane, who would never turn down a house-hunting excursion, came along for the fun. Despite our agent's good intentions, the house was isolated, far away from any metro stop, and it contained at least a half dozen small staircases, making it difficult for Old Mosely to scoot around.

As long as we were out and about, however, Danny said that there was one more house he wanted us to see. So, he drove us into a small subdivision in north Silver Spring near the town of Wheaton. Modest red brick ramblers shared quiet tree lined streets with a lesser number of modern, custom-built colonials. The ramblers were the original homes in this community built in the 50's. At first glimpse, these houses looked nearly identical to me, like stepping into a Brady Bunch set. "If we come home a little tipsy," I said, "we might not be able to remember which house is ours."

When the car came to a stop, however, my hopes lifted. We were parked in front of the one house in the neighborhood that looked different from all the rest: a gray/blue split level that brought to mind an old-fashioned farmhouse. It was landscaped in the front with bushes, shrubbery, and a variety of colorful flowers, and in the back with white and pink dogwoods. We agreed that Jane and Terri should go in for a quick look to see whether it would be worth the extra effort to bring me in. As with each of our recent house hunting outings, we brought along my manual wheelchair so that I could be lifted up or down stairs where necessary. Now, I waited in the car. Within minutes Jane rushed over to me.

"We have to find a way to get you inside this house," she said. She guessed that if we could overcome the accessibility dilemma, the house would be perfect for us. It backed out to the woods, was close to bike and jogging trails, rolling distance from a supermarket, and within a mile of a metro stop. But, as Jane recognized, there were obstacles I'd face in the nature of stairs.

"There are two steps to the front porch," Jane explained. "Once you get inside the house there's a tiny foyer. You then have a short staircase up to the main level and there also are stairs going down."

"I think I can leave the chair with you and scoot up the stairs backwards," I said.

In real estate jargon such a house is called a "split-foyer." There was a back door entrance to the lower floor, but no pathway leading to it. Getting me inside wouldn't be so easy, but I was game to try. I didn't realize that my effort would soon lead to an awkward moment.

I transfer from the car into the wheelchair, and then our agent helps Terri carry me in the chair over the flagstone steps to the front porch. Terri helps me out of the chair onto the first step. I sit there with my back to the entrance. Then I lift myself up the second step to the porch and push myself backward toward the front door. Thank goodness that at least my arms were gaining strength. I couldn't have managed even this meager feat one or two months earlier.

Once inside the house, I push myself up the five steps to the living room on my butt. The owner's agent is showing the house to several other couples. Jane observes a scowl on the agent's face as I maneuver myself up the stairs. Like a drenching rain on the Fourth of July, I'm ruining a good party. Danny must sense the awkwardness of the moment as well. To his credit, he isn't backing down. Terri wheels me around the main floor and then helps me into a chair in the living room. Now, I too can detect a look of annoyance from the owner's agent. If she could have her wish we would all just disappear into thin air.

The house was spacious and generally accessible. Indeed, it had just about everything we could want. The living room, in particular, reminded me of a great room in a ski lodge, with cathedral ceilings and glass doors opening onto a back deck that spanned the length of the house. The deck looked out to the woods of Sligo Creek Park. A gas fireplace separated the two glass door entrances. As for the lower level, I'd have to be content to let the others describe it to me. Terri told me that it had a family room with a wood-burning fireplace, several bedrooms that could alternatively serve as home offices, and sufficient space to house

Jessica and Daniel until they could afford their own place. We were sold.

To the amazement of the owners' agent, the next day we presented an offer to buy the house, contingent upon an accessibility inspection to be conducted within the following 48 hours. Would it be feasible to put in an elevator? How much other work would have to be done to make the entire house accessible to me?

The owners accepted our offer based on our willingness to allow a leaseback for two months. The leaseback would afford us time to pack up and sell our Connecticut Avenue condo, as well as to arrange construction work on the Wheaton house.

The inspection revealed that an elevator could be installed in the house, but not at the front entrance foyer. Instead, the elevator would go from the workshop behind the family room in the lower level of the house up to the kitchen. We'd also need a path leading from the driveway in front, circling around the side of the house to the back entrance. This wouldn't be difficult, although construction of the path would require shaving back the branches of a beautiful large pine tree. Such tradeoffs, we figured, are sometimes a necessary compromise. Also, the master bathroom would have to be reconfigured with a wider doorway to allow Old Mosely access and the shower enlarged to be handicap friendly.

The combined work would cost a substantial amount. The elevator alone would come to $17,500. Our hope was that in a relatively short time I might not need an elevator. Nevertheless, as a good friend put it, if you spend the money, you can be sure that someday you won't need the elevator. I adopted this superstitious notion wholeheartedly.

19 The Way Back

In early December 2001, soon after the San Diego trip when we were still living in the condo, Billie announced during therapy that it was time for me to walk with a four-pronged cane instead of the walker. "I think you are ready to progress," she said.

She placed the walker in front of the lift chair and ushered me to the edge of the kitchen. From there I would begin to walk across the living room, and down the narrow hall to my bedroom. She glanced at her watch; she would time me. I was terrified:

I step into my walker and move over to where Billie stands waiting. A moment of dread. I'm a child being told to swim on my own for the first time. Butterflies flutter from my stomach to my heart. Is it fear of falling or fear of failure? Sure, negotiating the lobby stairs had become old hat, but there I could place my hands on both railings, while Billie stayed right behind me with one hand on my safety belt and the other ready to prevent me from going down. But this is uncharted territory. Why can't she just leave me alone to perform my usual regimen of exercises, the routine with which I've become comfortable? Because, I suppose, that wouldn't lead to the improvement I so covet. If my nerves don't respond, I'll have only physical therapy of this sort to rely on to function independently. So I have no choice. I better give it my all, or reconcile myself to a sedentary life. And if I choose that, I'll be letting down everyone, especially Terri who's stood by me for better or worse. And, I'd be letting down myself. "You are who you are." Isn't that what I've been told? So, who am I?

I'd been forced to grapple with this question more than I'd have liked over this long, strange journey. I was never the heroic type, not one to step forward and take on risky ventures or difficult challenges. To the contrary, when stationed in right field in high school I'd pray the ball didn't get hit my way, or I'd sit in the back of the class and hope I didn't get called on, fretful that I'd fumble that tricky algebra or science question. I entered law school at the time the Vietnam War was escalating, fearing not a bad grade so much as a high lottery number that would make me vulnerable to the draft. During much of my marriage to Sylvia I'd avoid controversy if at all possible in order to keep the peace, choosing the path of least resistance. Any financial investments I made had to be safe. If someone had told me years ago that I'd face a crippling illness, I wouldn't have believed I could pull through it without falling apart or being overcome with anger and despair.

I may have changed over the years but that wasn't something about which I was particularly aware. In fact, I think people don't often notice change they undergo until others make them aware of it. At least it's been that way with me. Only after friends and family convinced me that I would sink to the bottom if I persisted in staying in a bad marriage was I able to walk away. When a friend fixed me up with a blind date, I told the woman to look for a fortyish man, about 5 foot ten, with brown hair. I utterly forgot my hair had turned gray years before. My date felt it necessary to call my attention to that as she'd had difficulty spotting me.

When Sylvia died, I was thrust into the role of single parent to a learning disabled child, a role I took on without hesitation. When Terri came around I knew she was right for me, not something I'd have likely understood in the past. And when our friend Bridgid said let's go to Africa and climb Kilimanjaro, instead of shying away from the challenge, this non-risk taker said sure. And so I tackled my first mountain, quite literally, with success. Now, my second mountain, the figurative one, loomed even larger, posing the greatest challenge of my life.

So what should I do? Plead with Billie to put off this daunting task for another day? "I'm too tired. I'm not ready." Or accept the challenge. "Let's give it a go." Who am I?

Billie pulls the walker aside and places the cane in my right hand. I grip it like a lifeline while she stands behind me, her left hand on my safety belt, her right hand on the cane. I guess she isn't pushing me into the deep end of the pool, not quite yet.

"Now, move the cane," she says.

She helps me move the cane about one foot ahead. "Now the left foot, bring it so that it is even with the cane. Now the right foot, a half step behind the left." We move this way, slowly across the living room floor to the narrow hallway leading to the bedrooms. "Bend your knees slightly," Billie instructs. Move the cane, I repeat to myself. Now left, now right. Slowly, slowly, or polé, polé, as the porters kept reminding us on Kilimanjaro. It seems an eternity.

"Now, turn to the left down the hall," Billie says as she guides my hand.

I'm sweating bullets but gaining confidence with each step. To calm myself I glance at the wall hangings as I go by. Enlarged photos we'd taken of African safari animals steel my gaze as I maneuver down the hall. We pass Jessica's room and enter mine. We made it there in 15 or 20 minutes, a trip that would take any able person about 10 seconds. I collapse on the bed with a sigh of relief: it's done, it's done. Now I can relax and do my regular exercises.

Billie and I continued to incorporate this routine into my twice-weekly sessions in the coming weeks. The time it took me to travel from the kitchen entrance to my bedroom improved steadily. Within one or two months I was walking, first with Terri and then on my own, down the eighth floor corridor outside our apartment. I would stay close to the wall, occasionally reaching out to touch it for security like a novice skater clinging to the sides of the skating rink. I believed and hoped that my peripheral nerves were connecting with my quad muscles and hamstrings at long last. By now, far more than eighteen months had passed since my initial hospitalization. Better late than never. Perhaps once again, the doctors' predictions would prove wrong, only this time to my benefit.

In early spring, Billie escorted me outdoors for the first time. First we'd work the alley in back of our building. This was the alley that separated the rear of the building from the small park where two years earlier I'd sat on a bench reading, waiting for Terri to return from her errands. That was when I learned I could no longer walk, even with the help of my walker. That was the day I entered the hospital only to come home in a wheelchair several weeks later. The bench was still there in the same place.

This was also the alley where I had taught Jessica to ride a bike. Now I was re-learning how to walk. I suppose turnabout is fair play. Several neighbors from the building gave me a thumbs-up, stopping to commend me on my perseverance and progress. I enjoyed the attention and show of support.

After I mastered the alley, Billie, Terri and I ventured around the block, circling the building. These excursions took about a half hour. Whenever I came to an uneven step, I'd bend my knees slightly and take the step very slowly. Every crack in the sidewalk resembled the Grand Canyon.

That first excursion to the hospital when I could no longer walk without collapsing to the ground had been in April 2000. Now it was March 2002. My progress had been as tedious as groundwater flowing uphill, but finally, finally, it seemed to be picking up. "Where would it all lead?" Billie didn't have the answers, but she was optimistic and ever so persistent.

Billie wanted to see if I could step down from a curb during one of our outings. "Oh my, he can't do that," Terri gasped. Billie took my arm and helped me step down from the sidewalk. Her assessment of this effort was to wait awhile and try it again another day. Terri was more optimistic about the future. She predicted that by mid-summer I'd be ready to walk several blocks down Connecticut Avenue to our favorite Chinese restaurant where we had dined the night before I first entered the hospital. Now that would be a triumphant return. Ray, the owner, might even treat me to a free egg roll. Or better still, a gin and tonic.

In April, we received an invitation to a wedding ceremony from good friends whom we had introduced. Adam worked in my office while Quynh had worked with Terri. We anticipated that many colleagues from each office would attend. The last wedding I'd attended, I had taken Old Mosely onto the dance floor. Terri was good-natured and cautiously swung along with Old Mosely and me. People were amused, impressed, and careful to steer clear of us. We'd had fun, but that routine quickly got old. At the coming ceremony, with so many people we knew bound to be present, I resolved that I'd dance for real.

I had never in my life been much of a dancer. In New York, growing up, I'd been forced to go to Viola Wolfe Dancing School in mid-town Manhattan. All the boys dressed in jackets and ties, wore white gloves, drank fruit punch, and were each instructed to bow following a dance number. We danced the Lindy, Cha-Cha, and Mambo, among other numbers that were hot in the 50's. What we called multiplication dances assured that I couldn't get away with sitting on the sidelines all evening. When the music stopped, a dancing couple would break up and each would select a different partner from the sidelines. The experience was painful as I was quite shy.

Later in life I dated a woman who liked to dance, so at her insistence I took instruction in swing dancing at the Spanish Ballroom at Glen Echo Park, close to D.C. I must have taken several beginning swing lessons without ever graduating to the next level. Eventually, I grasped the basic steps, but never quite mastered the art of leading. I was afraid they'd pin my picture to the entrance with a diagonal slash through it.

Nevertheless, I was determined to dance at our friends' wedding as a show of my improved mobility. To that end, I enlisted Billie's help. After a few sessions, I could place each hand on my wife's shoulders, much as I'd done for swim therapy. We could shuffle back and forth and sideways. This was a start. "I can dance as well as ever," I quipped, and I wasn't far off the mark.

We took Old Mosely to the wedding celebration in May, as I remained utterly dependent on my old friend for getting around in any meaningful way. But, with so many of my work friends around, I decided to walk into the reception room upright with my four-pronged cane. I wanted to show off. I was glad to find several former colleagues there who I hadn't seen in several years. However, because these people hadn't seen me during my illness, I could sense in some a reaction of shock or sadness. They'd been told about my condition, undoubtedly, but they hadn't actually observed me. I assured everyone that I was on the mend. Those friends who had endured my struggle along with me applauded my progress. This is what I'd hoped for. This is why I wanted to dance.

The vast ballroom was packed with large round tables each seating 10-12 people. The dinner table where Terri, Jessica and I were sitting was at the opposite end of the room from the dance floor, so getting there from our table required a certain degree of agility. I chose Jessica to be my first guinea pig. I placed my hands on her shoulders and we weaved our way around several dining tables until we reached the far edge of the dance floor. There, we shuffled back and forth with an occasional side turn. I was back at Viola Wolfe, the dancing school of my childhood, relearning the basic steps.

After a little rest, warmed by champagne, I danced with Terri. Now I was gaining confidence. But, I didn't dare try my moves on anyone else, not yet. Maybe I'd be ready to dance the night away at the next celebration. By evening's end, I felt that this adventure had shown a level of progress. I was on the way back. I felt invigorated and vowed to redouble my efforts in therapy. Like a much-coveted oasis in the desert, I could sense the road to recovery around the next bend.

Shortly after our friends' wedding, I think it was in June, I accompanied my wife on what was, for her, a business trip to Puerto Rico. We stayed at the Caribe Hilton. The hotel had a large pool divided into separate sections, with cascading water and a swim up bar. Swimming had become a favorite activity as it masked the full extent of my disability. I steered my rental chair down a ramp from the higher patio to the pool area. With Terri's help, I shifted onto a lounge chair close to the deep end of the pool. Then I sat up on the edge of the chair, eased myself down to the ground, pushed myself forward on my butt to the pool's edge, and splashed into the pool from a sitting position. Without missing a beat, I swam back and forth the length of the pool for a half hour. I was reminded now of why I had longed to move to San Diego: water and warm climate. If the world was filled with water, I'd be just about as mobile as the next guy.

After she'd finished work for the day, Terri met me at the pool, put on her bathing suit, and joined me for happy hour at the pool bar. We ordered rum punches, adult style. The bartender obliged. We drank several rum punches, we smooched, we toasted to my continued recovery. And then we smooched some more, long slurpy kisses, like in days gone by when I'd been courting her. Then we staggered upstairs to our room for a romantic interlude before dinner. The future looked as bright as it had in quite a while.

When we returned from Puerto Rico, we began in earnest the arduous process of packing up the apartment in preparation for our move to the house we had just bought in suburbia.

20 Descending the Mountain

Over that summer, while we contracted for the work on our new home and zealously planned our move, my walking steadily improved. At first, I took the four-pronged cane on my walks up and down the hallways at home and at the office. Then, one day, when I felt relatively strong, I leaned the cane outside the door of my apartment and shuffled down the hall without it, practically hugging the wall for security, as I'd done when I first started walking with the cane.

When Daniel, Jessica's high school sweetheart, came out of the apartment into the hall, I said, "Look Daniel, no cane."

Daniel is a young man of few words, never effusive in his praise. But now, his face lit up and he beamed. "Look at you, Michael. I'll bet you'll be walking normal in a few weeks. All that hard work is paying off."

"Maybe. But I better not count my Whitetails before they're cooked." Daniel, a true blue red neck and proud of it, takes his deer hunting seriously.

Before long, I was regularly taking my daily walks without cane or walker. Concurrently, my distances for set times on the recumbent bike increased significantly week-by-week. This progress wasn't solely the result of physical therapy. At last, I concluded, my nerves were reconnecting with my muscles and the muscles, in turn, were responding. It had now been over two years since my initial hospitalization. The eighteen-month outer limit on improvement, which had haunted me like a stubborn ghost, had turned out to be overplayed. I can't reasonably blame my doctors. Medical science was not advanced far enough for anyone to predict the outcome of my illness with precision. Dr. Sherman, my internist, had cautioned at the outset that treating my condition and predicting its outcome, would be tantamount to practicing voodoo medicine.

It was around this time that Dr. Sherman relayed to me his theory about my appendicitis, that my sudden medical emergency a year ago may have shifted the focus of the antibodies, the demonic warriors of my immune system, away from their misguided war on my nerves. Instead, they were redirected to an urgent defense of my body from the bacteria produced by the ruptured appendix. Although speculative, the timing of events gives credence to Dr. Sherman's theory.

During the first year of my illness, from my hospitalization in April 2000 until my appendix ruptured in late February 2001, the treatments I received in the hospital and afterward, while not making me better, possibly kept me from getting worse. The mild relapses that I suffered around the winter holidays of 2000—01 may have been held at bay by the prednisone. My condition held steady then until my appendectomy. Several months after that hospitalization, before our San Diego trip, I finally began to gain upper body strength. Using my arms, I was able for the first time to transfer myself from my wheelchair to my lift chair or to my bed. This didn't happen all at once. The nerves must have been regenerating for several months, possibly beginning their slow, unimpeded journey following the appendicitis. Then, starting in the spring of 2002 and continuing throughout that summer, my legs gradually gained strength. The nerves, of course, had a longer distance to travel in my legs, which explains the added delay.

Viewed through this lens, there seems to be support for Dr. Sherman's hypothesis. But who knows?

Of course, I still couldn't tell how much I'd recover. My foot balance remained unsteady. My distal muscles (the ones that are most distant from my torso and control my hands and feet) were still weak: I couldn't wiggle my toes, flex my ankles, or flex my fingers. Foot balance, however, was my biggest problem. I couldn't stand still for more than a few seconds without having to adjust my stance. I needed a cane coupled with a helping hand to step up and down curbs. But still, with the aid of my ankle flexion orthotics and a straight cane, I could once again venture outdoors on foot. I now had sound reason to hope for and expect a substantial recovery.

I had climbed to within sight of the summit, but would I complete the descent to base camp?

With James leading the way, our spirited group, giddy from having reached the roof of Africa, begins to descend Kilimanjaro by way of the steep Mweka trail. Instead of re-circling the summit the way we'd come up, we'll head straight down this steeper route. Mweka would've made for a difficult route to the top but presented a practical alternative for a fast descent.

Now that it's daylight, I search all around the snow and rocks for the carcass of the leopard that Hemingway had said was found on these higher slopes. A lasting mystery as to why this creature had climbed so high, and so far out of its habitat. Indeed, as I look around, I see only the snow and rocks and pebbles that mountaineers call scree, but nothing on which to feed. What was it searching for? There is abundant wildlife on Kilimanjaro on the lower slopes where vegetation flourishes. But the mountain terrain is so vast it would take enormous luck to spy any, especially the elusive and solitary leopard.

I'm not athletic, so I spend much of the first day of our descent sliding downhill on my backside. I'm fit enough to maintain a steady pace uphill, but unlike your average soccer player, I'm not agile enough to scramble headlong downhill on my feet. So I take it slowly, cautiously easing myself down loose scree and dirt, holding onto boulders or whatever else is around that I can grab. Lisa and Ray are well ahead of Terri and me, and before long Terri runs on ahead of me. James lags behind, keeping a wary eye on both of us. There's no one to chat with, but that is just as well as we are exhausted. We just want to get to our last night's camp and collapse in our tents. Maybe, if the mountain gods take pity on us, we'll even get some sleep.

I welcome the sight of the brown tents that the porters have set up in anticipation of our arrival. Camp tonight is at 10,000 feet, just above the rain forest. Steep and slippery, the rain forest was my greatest nemesis on the way up and is likely to be even more of a challenge on the way down. I dread the morning but am too tired now to worry about it. The porters bring us tea and nuts followed by a dinner of shredded beef and rice. Not long after dinner I slip into my sleeping bag and drift off, as does Terri.

I sleep on and off, in fits and starts. At daybreak I arise feeling grumpy. Our tents are small so I must be careful to stoop down low to enter or exit. I've passed this test so far. I have to pee awful bad so I rush out to find a private spot to claim as a toilet. As I leave I feel the roof of the tent collapse on top of me. I'm tangled in the canvass and have to fight my way out. I hear laughter inside. "It was just a matter of time," Terri calls out. Ray and Lisa and the porters are amused by my mishap, but with less than a good night's sleep, I'm not.

The morning air is crisp and cool. We wash our faces in the bowl of lukewarm water that the porters have brought to our tent, and then join the others for a breakfast of eggs, toast, and cereal. After breakfast, we set out on our final leg of the journey.

After hiking a short way we find ourselves, once again, tackling the rain forest. This time, I'm mentally prepared for the worst. Despite the mud, I willfully spend most of the day sliding down the steepest segments of the trail on my butt. I know I'll be filthy by the end of the day anyway, so what the hell. When, after about six hours, we emerge at the gate entrance leading to Mweka Village, I'm bathed in dirt and grime and sweat. But so are we all.

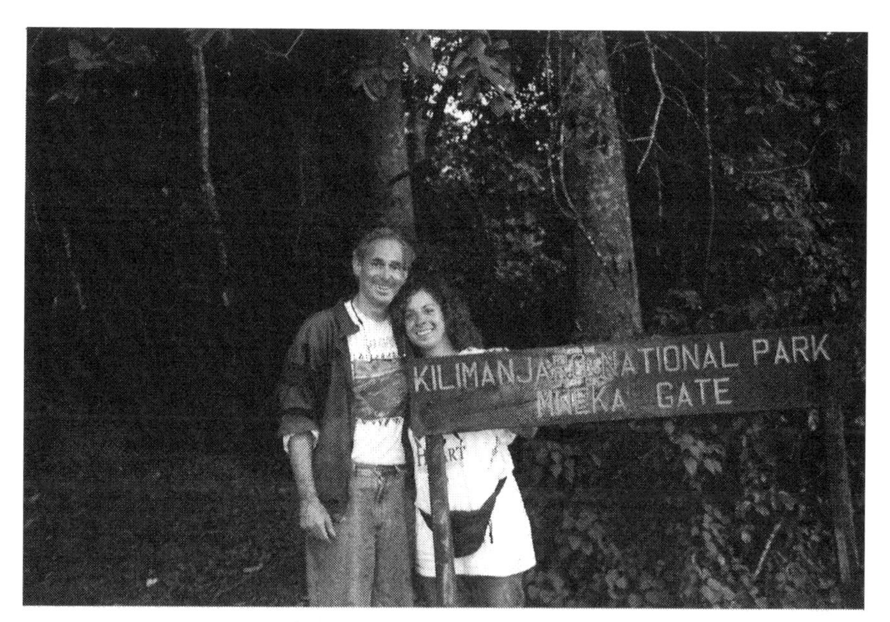

Terri and Michael at Mweka Gate having
safely descended Kilimanjaro

Several weeks after Terri and I returned home, we received a package from Ray and Lisa. Inside, we found various reminders of the trip. Among these were several enlarged panoramic photos from the climb, a couple of power bars, a liter of bottled water, and a roll of toilet paper. Great remembrances.

I don't harbor any notion that climbing Kilimanjaro was some remarkable athletic feat, the equivalent, for example, of conquering the seven summits or sailing around the South Pole or running a sub-three hour marathon. Thousands reach the summit of Kilimanjaro every year. But for me, and I'm sure for Terri, our successful venture marked a special personal achievement. Setting a goal beyond anything I'd ever imagined for myself, and persevering to achieve it, was an accomplishment of which I could be proud.

In trekking up Kilimanjaro did I use up my mobility, as my cousin Judy would later claim? Did absorbing the rarified atmosphere potentially lead to my neuropathy, as Dr. Sherman would suggest? I doubt it. I knew that high altitude could lead to toxic neuropathy, but in such cases the symptoms are more immediate and generally subside upon descent to lower altitudes. That's why the neurologists at George Washington didn't think our trip to Africa caused my condition: the four-month lapse between our return and when my first symptoms cropped up made any connection between the two way too attenuated. Also, little is known about the effect of high altitude on the immune system. Someday we'll know more, but not yet.

What I do know is that Terri and I set out to accomplish what was for us a challenging goal. In persevering to the end, we may have prepared ourselves for future challenges. For the next mountain.

The prior owners moved out of the Wheaton house at the end of July, as planned, and construction on the house began the first week of August. We planned our move for the Labor Day weekend.

The master bathroom was outfitted with a full size shower complete with a pull down seat and bars on two sides. Instead of two narrow doorways, the bathroom now had one wider doorway that allowed Old Mosely access to the shower, provided its driver used caution. We had constructed a paved path that led to the rear entrance of the house, where a French door was installed to replace the sliding glass door that had been there before. The elevator, which would become a showpiece for our guests, especially the toddler set, was placed in the downstairs workshop, as planned. A square of the kitchen floor above was cut so the elevator could rise into the kitchen. As the elevator made its upward climb into the kitchen, it lifted the cut square of floor, which then became the elevator ceiling. Incredibly, given the peculiar nuances of construction schedules, the house was ready to receive us on schedule.

We took a week off around Labor Day to accomplish the move and settle into our new home. I decided that the week of the move would mark a milestone in my road to recovery. When I returned to the office the following week, I'd leave Old Mosely behind. I phoned Alice, the office Manager.

"Hi Alice. Could you put in an order for a desk chair, please.

One that rolls, and has a high back. I'm not going to use my wheelchair any more." I knew that finally I could rise up from a stationary chair, so long as I could push down on the desk to help me up. The thick carpet would help keep a rolling chair somewhat stationary as I pushed down on the desk to help me get up onto my feet.

"Okay, Michael. I'll order a chair as you like, but it may take a week to arrive. You better keep using your wheelchair for now."

"No, that's okay. I'll take any old chair until the new one comes." I was adamant. Now that I was mobile, I fully intended to abandon all badges of my disability except those that remained essential.

My first day back at the office without Old Mosely was an emotional one for me. When I walked into the conference room for our weekly staff meeting with just a cane for support, I was greeted by the applause of my colleagues. "You deserved that applause," Terri remarked when I told her about it later that evening, and she gave me a monster hug.

For two and a half years, from April 2000 until Labor Day 2002, I'd been wheelchair bound, needing help in just getting up from the chair, and in all facets of daily life. "I am who I am," I'd been told. Had this experience told me who I was? Maybe just a little.

Terri and I had met this challenge together, just as we'd climbed Kilimanjaro together. I now knew what I was capable of achieving with Terri beside me. Alone, I'm not sure. But that wasn't the challenge that I'd faced. Also, I'd been lucky, in a sense. With CIDP, I was told I'd get better. Sure, the road was bumpy and it wasn't over yet. But how would I have fared with an illness where I'd get worse and remain incapacitated? I don't know.

Two and a half years. Thirty months. Indeed, Terri and I had been in a marathon, just as we'd been warned, not a sprint. I'd keep on racing as far as I could, but by now I'd pushed through the wall at mile twenty. So long as Terri was by my side, rooting me on, I'd damn well finish the race.

21 The Road Ahead

Today Old Mosely sits in the laundry room of our Wheaton home, its battery long dead, discarded objects such as a torn rug and broken hangars piled on its seat. Like the grownup boy in *Puff the Magic Dragon*, the chair's master has outgrown his use for it.

After we moved into the Wheaton house, we kept Old Mosely in our bedroom on the main floor. Eventually, I stopped using my chair except when I showered. Although the bathroom doorway was wide enough for me to maneuver the chair close enough to the shower to allow me to transfer to the pull-down seat, if I failed to guide the chair just right, it damaged the freshly painted walls. Such mishaps occurred regularly. Before long, I stopped using Old Mosely altogether. At first, I left the chair in the bedroom. Eventually, the battery went dead. Sometime later, Terri guided it manually, by the way of the elevator, to the utility room downstairs. There it stays, unwanted and unneeded, a vivid reminder of the way things were.

I used the elevator for several weeks, but gradually I found it simpler to use the stairs. I grabbed onto the railings or walls to help pull myself up or to balance myself going down. The elevator was a novelty and came in handy now and then, but it became a chore to use regularly, so I used it less and less. We enjoyed demonstrating how it worked. Small children, in particular, were mesmerized by it. Today, our cats' food and water bowls sit on the square floor of the kitchen intended for the elevator. We have to move these things to allow the elevator to come up. Rarely do we need to do this. Did spending the $17,500 aid my recovery? If so, I don't regret a penny.

Billie continued her sessions with me, one day a week at first, and then every other week. She said the focus of my therapy should be on walking. Foot drop was now my most serious physical problem. Walking around the house without shoes and orthotics proved tricky at first, but soon I was able to hobble around in just socks, all the while being careful to lift my feet high with each step. Terri called this my "pelican walk." Stumbling and tripping was always a hazard, but I didn't want to wear shoes every waking minute. By now, I was using a straight cane.

Over the 2002 winter holidays, Billie failed to show up for one of our scheduled sessions. At first this didn't concern us as she'd been in the habit of cancelling sessions without notice when she was called out of town. But in the past she'd always phone us after the fact to re-schedule. This time, however, she didn't call and our efforts to contact her proved fruitless. My hunch was that she was summoned back home to Uganda to care for her ailing mother. In any event, we never saw or heard from her again, and our periodic efforts to reach her invariably ended in disappointment. As I think back on this time, I know she thought she'd done all she could for me and likely felt it was time to move on. Perhaps she had a psychological block about saying good-bye for keeps. Still, her disappearance was a puzzle because we had always been on good terms. We would miss her.

I kept to the regimen that Billie had designed for me. Eventually, I stopped using my cane in the house, and left it in the umbrella stand by the front door. I only used it on my outdoor walks. I needed it for stamina and curbs. At first, Terri or Jessica would accompany me outside. By the spring of 2003, however, particularly on nice days, I would take unaccompanied walks in the neighborhood, sometimes hobbling along for two miles or more. Slowly and steadily, *polé, polé*. As my walking continued to improve and I could better navigate curbs, I stopped using a cane altogether. I found that not taking a cane on walks or errands left both my hands free to carry groceries or other stuff.

Around this time, I decided to reclaim my driver's license. The last time I'd driven a car was in April 2000, shortly before I entered the hospital when I could no longer walk. Terri had exchanged my license for a handicap placard with the understanding that I could get the license back within four months without having to take any tests, assuming I had a certification from my doctor that I could drive. I'd been hopeful then that I'd get well enough within the four-month time frame to be able to drive, but that was not to be. Now, three years later, I was ready. Terri took me to a large parking area in nearby Wheaton Park. I found that using the foot pedals was difficult and tiring. We opted for hand controls. Like any number of automobile companies, Subaru contributes to the cost of having such devices installed, asking only for medical documentation and the purchase agreement. The fellow who installed the controls had me drive around my neighborhood and before long I was able to pass the road test and reclaim my license.

Being able to drive again was liberating, allowing me to assert a greater degree of independence. Also, I could go places for work such as rural areas or small towns where taxi transport wasn't feasible. I was back in the saddle.

Now that I could move on my own, Terri and I wasted no time in planning trips abroad. Terri got so excited about our new freedom she almost forgot to renew her passport. "When does yours expire, Michael?" she asked. Oops.

In the years following our move to the Wheaton house, we ventured into Turkey, France, Southeast Asia, and Guatemala, among other places. When traveling outside of the United States, I would always bring my cane to help me navigate the cobbled streets and steep curbs of foreign cities. Mountain climbing may be off the agenda, but foreign travel is in my blood.

In Istanbul we hiked from the Blue Mosque in the old quarter, across the Golden Horn, and uphill to the Istiklal Caddesi, a pedestrian thoroughfare in one of Istanbul's newer sections. We paused along the way to climb the several flights of steps to the top of the medieval Galata Tower. We took a ride on a tour boat off the Aegean coast, stopping at various coves to swim. The clear turquoise water beckoned. I was not to be denied. I jumped off the boat into the water at several of these stops and frolicked to my heart's content. When it was time to get back in the boat, I climbed the ladder with Terri right behind me, guiding my feet as I lifted them one rung to the next. Billie would have been proud.

In Paris we walked from one end of the city to the other, picnicking in the Luxembourg Gardens or the Tuileries. Paris is best explored on foot and this we did with relish. We found no shortage of cafes or park benches when I needed a rest. I'm sure we put in at least six miles each day traversing the city's colorful neighborhoods.

One day, from our small hotel in the Latin Quarter, we walked across the Seine to Notre Dame, and along the right bank to the Louvre. After a couple of hours in the museum, we continued our tour, ending up browsing through the food specialty shops around the Place de Madeleine. After picking up a couple of jars of mustard, we headed back to our hotel, stopping along the way for cappuccino. Quite a hike.

In Cassis, a picturesque harbor with a small sandy beach on the southern coast of France, I plunged into the Mediterranean Sea. For me, going into the water at any beach is easier than getting out, although I continue to improve at both. On the beach at Cassis, I took Terri by the hand and in we went, straddling the waves until the water was deep enough to float. When we decided it was time to return to the beach, Terri struggled to help me stand up and keep my balance. I kept tumbling backward into the swirling waves. "Hold onto my shoulders," Terri instructed, "and follow me to the beach." I tried, but along came a menacing wave that knocked us both down. Two lovely young women, both topless, saw our dilemma and rushed to my aid. (This was France after all).

"May we help you, monsieur?"

"*Mais oui*." After all, how could I refuse their offer to help? I guess there are times when a disability has its rewards.

In Laos, Vietnam and Cambodia, I got on and off more boats

than I could count, and climbed up steep river embankments to primitive tribal villages, usually with a helping hand from our caring guides. The people in those countries are as friendly as can be, and there was nowhere that I couldn't go thanks to their eagerness to help.

In Guatemala, I climbed the makeshift stairways of two ancient temples at the Mayan ruins in Tikal. I didn't want to miss out on the sweeping views of the jungle from up high. I left my cane with the guide and pulled myself up the hundreds of steps using the rope handrails. The resulting blisters were worth the views and the challenge. "Bravo," one lady called out to me as I made my way down. I always appreciate such thoughtful and well-intentioned acknowledgement.

Most of my days, of course, were spent at the Justice Department or on the road for depositions or witness interviews and meetings on complex toxic tort cases. Following one such meeting that I chaired, one of our expert witnesses pulled me aside. "Michael," he asked, "now that you're on the way to a full recovery, are you gratified that you've been given this window into what it's like to be truly disabled?"

I had to think about this. "I'm not sure," I said. "I guess I'd like to first know that my eventual recovery will be complete. Then, maybe."

Indeed, I appreciated what he was saying. I'd gained a feel for the frustration involved in being confined to a wheelchair. I now understood the importance of cut curbs and how maddening it is when cars park smack in front of them. I sensed the fear of being thwarted from riding the metro in the event an elevator was out-of-service. I'd learned the hard way that speed bumps were not obstacles to be trifled with. And I now understood how much the commitment of caregivers—nurses, therapists and loved ones—made it possible to survive, yet, at the same time, how vulnerable it feels to need the help of a spouse or friends, even strangers, to simply function in the world.

But would I go through two and a half wheelchair-bound years again to learn these lessons? To better empathize with others who were similarly impaired? The truth is I'm not that heroic. As I thought back on my experience, the most frightening thing was the uncertainty, not knowing whether I'd ever recover or to what extent. And that fear remained. While I'd come a long way back, I remained hobbled with a full recovery unlikely. If given a choice, I expect I'd rather be planning our next trekking adventure.

I continued to see my neurologist, Dr. Richardson, once every six months, mainly so he could chart my progress. He'd administer his standard neurologic exam, ranking the strength of each muscle group from trace (almost no strength) to five (normal strength). With each visit, for a time, the strength of certain muscles showed slight improvement. Dr. Richardson also checked for changes in the sensation in my upper and lower extremities. The distal regions—hands, feet, ankles—continued to display sensory loss. To this day my hands and feet feel stiff, although the buzzing in my feet has subsided.

After a couple of years, when it seemed I'd reached a fairly even plateau, I stopped making the appointments with Dr. Richardson. There didn't seem to be any point in going through the same battery of tests when I had little reason to expect any significant change in the results. My dorsiflexion wasn't improving, however, the orthotics allowed me to walk pretty good distances.

Even though I'd reached a plateau, I continued to see functional improvement over time. My wrists strengthened to the point where I could open a corked bottle of wine—no insignificant achievement. I went back to George Washington Hospital as an outpatient in the spring of 2004 to update my physical therapy regimen. By then a deluxe new hospital had taken the place of the old one. I sought out the therapists with whom I'd worked. Unfortunately, Beth had left for work elsewhere and Michelle was on leave. Even so, I found a couple of staff members from the bad old days to whom I could boast about my improved condition.

The new regimen had me doing strengthening exercises for my arm and leg muscles three days a week. Six days a week, for a cardio work out, I would ride my recumbent bike for half an hour, alternating hard and easy days. I'd walk once or twice daily, covering up to two or three miles each day. This was not a strenuous routine, but I stuck to it rigidly and continue with it to this day.

Even today, my walking continues to get stronger and my new fitbit keeps me honest. Stairs remain difficult because ankle flexion is necessary to initiate a climb. I compensate by pushing and pulling myself using handrails. If I'm confronted with a set of narrow or steep stairs without railings, I need someone to lend me a hand.

Had my immune system shut down sooner, had the early treatments worked better, I suppose I might have made a fuller recovery. I don't know. I only know that I played the hand that I was dealt. I'm grateful to be able to function independently and especially to be walking on my own. Perhaps the distal muscles would have responded if the nerves had been permitted to complete their journey within eighteen months, unimpeded by setbacks. It's unlikely that I'll recover dorsiflexion, the muscles that allow the feet to flex upward, but my other muscles seem to compensate when I work consistently to strengthen them. At times folks who see me infrequently will comment on my improvement. I'm doing everything within my power to sustain this level of recovery for the rest of my days.

And Terri and I, having conquered two mountains together, are closer than ever before, ready to tackle our next, as yet-unknowable ascent.

About the Author

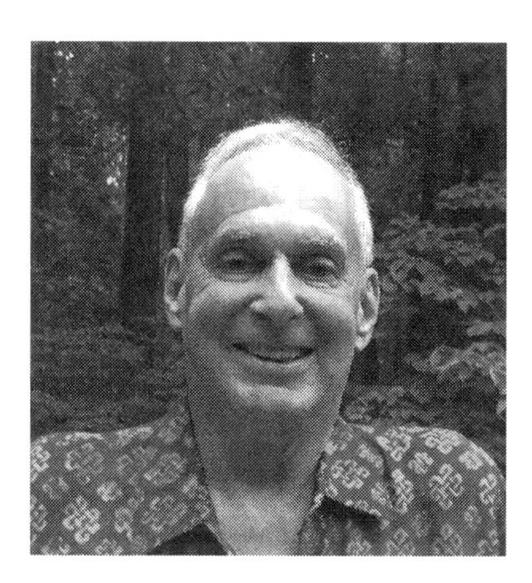

S. Michael Scadron lives in Silver Spring, MD, with his wife Terri and two rescue cats. A veteran Senior Trial Counsel with the U.S. Justice Department, Michael's passion for civil and human rights is expressed today by his advocacy for wrongfully convicted prisoners in the U.S. and abroad. He is also an award winning essayist whose non-fiction work has appeared in *The Christian Science Monitor*, in *Bethesda Magazine*, and on multiple travel websites. *Two Mountains* is his first full-length book.

An avid runner and trekker, Michael suffered a rare neurological disorder that rendered him quadriplegic just weeks after he reached the summit of Mount Kilimanjaro. Transformed from an active, vibrant 52-year old into a wheelchair-bound patient who needed assistance to feed, move, relieve, and clean his body, Michael faced a strange new world. His story recounts his climb up Kilimanjaro and his unprecedented ascent to walk again. It is an everyman story of inner strength, courage, and willingness to endure, as well as a recollection of the fond and funny moments that arise and comfort in the midst of fear.

Today Michael stays active, travels, and enjoys family and friends. He is most grateful for reclaiming the ability to walk and learning how to navigate life, albeit differently from any way he ever imagined.

70958238R00135

Made in the USA
Middletown, DE
18 April 2018